Effective Psychotherapy for Low-Income and Minority Patients

Effective Psychotherapy for Low-Income and Minority Patients

Frank X. Acosta, Ph.D.
University of Southern California School of Medicine
Los Angeles, California

Joe Yamamoto, M.D.
Neuropsychiatric Institute
University of California at Los Angeles
Los Angeles, California

and

Leonard A. Evans, Ph.D.
University of Southern California School of Medicine
Los Angeles, California

PLENUM PRESS • NEW YORK AND LONDON

Library of Congress Cataloging in Publication Data

Acosta, Frank X.
  Effective psychotherapy for low-income and minority patients.

  Bibliography: p.
  Includes index.
  1. Minorities—Mental health services—United States. 2. Poor—Mental health services—
United States. 3. Mental health services—United States. 4. Psychotherapy—Social aspects—
United States. I. Yamamoto, Joe. II. Evans, Leonard A. III. Title. [DNLM: 1. Minority groups.
2. Poverty. 3. Psychotherapy. 4. Community mental health services. WA 305 A185e]
RC451.5.A2A26 1982   362.2'042   82-9053
ISBN 0-306-40879-1   AACR2

© 1982 Plenum Press, New York
A Division of Plenum Publishing Corporation
233 Spring Street, New York, N.Y. 10013

Printed in the United States of America

Foreword

Psychotherapy involves a deep ethical commitment to self-knowledge, personal change, and mutual respect by both the therapist and the patient. Unfortunately, therapists have not always lived up to that commitment in understanding and treating low income and minority patients. Too often they lack the skills to understand and adjust to the patient's community and cultural experiences. The result has been ineffective and misguided treatment.

Effective Psychotherapy for Low-Income and Minority Patients is a handbook for psychotherapists interested and committed to correcting this situation and pursuing effective treatment strategies. This book is based on the author's ongoing innovative research project at the University of Southern California School of Medicine's Adult Psychiatric Outpatient Clinic. Located in East Los Angeles, the clinic serves this nation's largest Hispanic American community and has service commitments to residents of the central Los Angeles region. Over the years the authors have noted not only a marked need to improve mental health services, but also a need to make them more accessible to minority and low income patients. Generally these patients have very negative ideas about treatment of emotional problems. They typically react to treatment with skepticism: no one has really listened to them or understood them before—why should this therapist do so now? In describing this pessimism the authors discuss the need to listen to and respect each other. The authors outline how therapist and patient can explore emotional issues together in the context of the patient's social and cultural experiences. The authors explain the pressures which low income and minority patients face at home and in the workplace that make conventional mental health treatment ineffective and often harmful. They discuss many of the problems commonly faced by therapists, such as developing patient trust, and suggest effective therapeutic approaches.

I believe that *Effective Psychotherapy for Low-Income and Minority Patients* fills a critical gap in providing culturally sensitive mental health treatment. I recall from my earlier work as a public health educator visiting rural and urban communities in California that one refrain echoed throughout many of my visits: "no one listens to us very well." Now as a legislator sitting on the Labor, Health and Human Services and Education Appropriations Subcommittee, I have worked with dedicated health professionals, like Drs. Acosta, Yamamoto and Evans, to make our health establishment listen and listen well. This book tells us of the need to remain sensitive and respectful of each other's hopes and concerns. It teaches us never to lose sight of the importance of a caring society.

THE HONORABLE EDWARD R. ROYBAL

The United States House of Representatives
Washington, D.C.

Foreword

Despite the significant contributions made by the community mental health centers (CMHCs), major gaps still exist in those programs aimed at inadequately and inappropriately served groups. To a large extent, the CMHCs and the federal, state, and local governments have not responded adequately to the special needs of our pluralistic communities, especially within the major metropolitan areas. We have not taken seriously the fact that race and ethnicity are very important variables affecting treatment, outcome, and mental health services utilization.

A major problem is found in the continuing reliance on Western European tradition and practices in the treatment of low-income and minority patients. The "Anglo" approach to serving "people of color" has lost its credibility: It is in direct conflict with Hispanic, Asian, American Indian, and black culture. There is a commonality of harsh experiences that low-income and minority patients encounter as service users. They continue to be subjected to inferior treatment in mental health services delivery.

The disappointing experiences of racial and ethnic minorities in the delivery of mental health services, for example, negative outcomes, differential treatment, underutilization, and noncompliance, are referred to in numerous articles. However, there is virtually no textbook that specifically addresses positive approaches to psychotherapy for low-income blacks, Hispanics, Asians, Pacific Islanders, and whites. This textbook creatively fills the void. It represents new training perspectives that have applicability to a broad spectrum of disciplines—social work, psychology, psychiatry, nursing, sociology, and anthropology.

This book is aimed at helping practicing psychotherapists and providers of mental health services, as well as those in training, to be more knowledgeable and aware of the sociocultural characteristics of low-income and minority patients. Treatment guidelines and approaches are also presented to assist therapists in working with ethnic patients.

I believe that *Effective Psychotherapy for Low-Income and Minority Patients* will significantly stimulate future efforts to make mental health services not only more acceptable and appropriate but, more importantly, beneficial and cost-effective to the consumers.

Tom C. Owan

Chief, Services for Minorities Program
Mental Health Services Development Branch
Division of Mental Health Service Programs
National Institute of Mental Health
Rockville, Maryland

Preface

This book was written in response to the great need that exists in the mental health field for better understanding and guidelines for providing quality mental health services to patients from low-income and ethnic minority backgrounds. The number of minority, working-class, and poor people in the United States has traditionally been large. At present, very little clinically relevant information is available to psychotherapists to assist them in treating such patients. It is our hope that this book will prove useful to the clinician who works with these patients either in private practice or in mental health settings. It provides introductory information about the following low-income patient groups: Hispanic Americans, black Americans, Asian Americans, and Anglo-Americans. Of particular concern are the cultural, ethnic, economic, and psychological characteristics that describe these patients and can be used by therapists to understand them better as individuals. The book also specifies several potential problems that may be unique to these particular patients and a discussion of several therapeutic approaches that have proven effective with them.

The content material is likely to be of special interest to a variety of mental health care professionals including psychologists, psychiatrists, psychiatric nurses, social workers, police officers, educators, and counselors, who are called on regularly to evaluate and help persons with emotional disorders. This book is introductory in its scope and thus is well suited for both practitioners and students in these fields. It can also serve effectively as a basic review for those preparing for certifying and licensing examinations in psychology, psychiatry, nursing, and social work.

The format of this book facilitates learning because of its unique instructional design. Each chapter begins with an introduction that provides the reader with a conceptual frame of reference. Following the introduction, are the learning objectives, which highlight the essential points. These are followed by the content information necessary to enable a reader to achieve the stated objectives. Each content area is followed by a self-assessment exercise consisting of clinically oriented questions, which, if completed, will indicate learning progress. A closing paragraph summarizes the major content points of each chapter and is followed by a list of references that can be used to pursue the topic in greater depth.

The information presented here provides a solid foundation on which fundamental treatment skills can be developed. However, such information can only be transformed into clinical skills through actual practice.

The concluding chapter describes a special orientation program designed to prepare patients for therapy prior to their first therapeutic encounter. The information may be used by therapists or mental health centers as a model for developing similar materials to make psychotherapy more rewarding for both the low-income and the minority patient, as well as the therapist.

Development of this book was assisted by Grant MH 27899 from the National Institute of Mental Health, Mental Health Services Development Branch. We particularly wish to thank Howard Davis, Ph.D., Chief, Mental Health Services Development Branch, Division of Mental Health Service Programs, and Tom C. Owan, A.C.S.W., Chief, Services for Minorities Program, Mental Health Services Development Branch, Division of Mental Health Service Programs, for their continued encouragement and support of our work.

We also wish to thank Congressman Edward R. Roybal for his continued interest and encouragement of our work.

We further thank our editors, Sherwyn Woods, M.D. and Hilary Evans, for their technical guidance, review, and support of our work.

We are highly appreciative to Barbara Bass, M.S.W., Andrea K. Delgado, M.D., and Ching-piao Chien, M.D. for their important contributions.

Several of our colleagues reviewed drafts of our chapter manuscripts. We sincerely appreciated the critiques and suggestions made by Eligio R. Padilla, Ph.D., Alfonso Baez, M.D., Bertha Williams, Ph.D., Chester Pierce, M.D., Andrea K. Delgado, M.D., Gerald Dillingham, Ph.D., William M. Skilbeck, Ph.D., and Fritz Redlich, M.D.

Our book was developed with significant input from the psychiatric residents and clinical psychology interns who participated in our seminars. We are indebted to them for their important feedback and participation.

Our research project staff has been enthusiastically involved throughout the preparation of this book. We are grateful to Martha H. Cristo, Irma L. Diaz, Fabiola Gutierrez, Ana Lacabanne, and Sergio Martinez-Romero for their assistance.

FRANK X. ACOSTA
JOE YAMAMOTO
LEONARD A. EVANS

University of Southern California
Los Angeles, California

Contents

CHAPTER 1

Effective Psychotherapy for Low-Income and Minority Patients

Frank X. Acosta, Joe Yamamoto, Leonard A. Evans, and
Stuart A. Wilcox

CHAPTER 2

The Poor and Working-Class Patient

Joe Yamamoto, Frank X. Acosta, and Leonard A. Evans

CHAPTER 3

The Hispanic-American Patient

Frank X. Acosta and Leonard A. Evans

CHAPTER 4

The Black American Patient

Barbara A. Bass, Frank X. Acosta, and Leonard A. Evans

CHAPTER 5

On Being Black

Andrea K. Delgado

CHAPTER 6

Asian-American and Pacific-Islander Patients

Ching-piao Chien and Joe Yamamoto

CHAPTER 7

Putting It All Together

Leonard A. Evans, Frank X. Acosta, and Joe Yamamoto

CHAPTER 1

Effective Psychotherapy for Low-Income and Minority Patients

Frank X. Acosta, Joe Yamamoto, Leonard A. Evans, and Stuart A. Wilcox

INTRODUCTION

The poor, the working-class, or the minority person who needs psychotherapy is characteristically underserved by mental health establishments, which are primarily geared to the needs of middle- or upper-class and nonminority patients (Acosta, 1977; Sue, 1977; Yamamoto, James, & Palley, 1968). Therapists who make up the mental health establishments often lack the knowledge necessary to work effectively with minority populations and subgroups (President's Commission on Mental Health, 1978). Given this lack of knowledge and the existence of racism in the United States, it is not surprising that many mental health professionals have prejudicial attitudes toward minority groups, which can be manifested either in outright rejection or in the provision of less intensive, less interested, unenthusiastic care (Lorion, 1974). These patients will continue to be underserved until mental health professionals become better trained to deal with the unique problems of these patients more effectively.

Paradoxically, even professionals who are aware of their prejudices and who try to counter them in order to offer appropriate treatment for the *emotional problems* of minority and poor patients may at times fail to recognize the influence of the patient's social and environmental problems. Failure to take these into consideration is another reason why poor and minority patients are not well served.

1

Patients need to be met on their own grounds, their perceived needs and requests must be heard and understood, before remedies which make sense in the context of their social reality may be offered.

It is the purpose of this chapter to present an overview of the special problems that face psychotherapists in an outpatient clinic or mental health facility that serves significant numbers of poor, working-class, and minority patients and to describe some of the efforts which may be taken to help resolve these problems.

After completing this chapter and a corresponding group discussion session you should be able to:

1. Describe the characteristics of the poor, working-class, and minority patient that may affect the service they receive at a mental health facility
2. Describe the possible effects of certain characteristics of upper-middle-class therapists who are providing therapy for such patients
3. Discuss the major reasons patients have for coming to a mental health facility
4. Discuss the treatment issues important in a typical mental health facility
5. Recognize, encourage, and reinforce patient assertive statements

Please read the above learning objectives until you become familiar with the goals of this chapter; then continue reading the following section.

THE PATIENT–THERAPIST DYAD

Social and Cultural Factors

It is critical for therapists to be aware of their patients' sociocultural and ethnic backgrounds, that is, their ethnicity, social class, race, religion, and age, and how these factors influence both patients' psychological state and their degree of comfort in relating to the therapist. Members of minority or low-income groups face the special stress of discrimination and/or economic hardship that create problems not felt by nonminority or more affluent individuals. The extent to which the patient's values and perspectives coincide or conflict with the therapist's values may also be crucial to effective patient–therapist interaction. Typically, the educational process for psychotherapists does not include discussion of these variables. While it is true for most professions, it is of special importance that psychotherapists be aware of how their own backgrounds and experiences may enter into their dialogue with patients. Therapists should ask themselves what the similarities and differences between themselves and their patients are. They must anticipate the kind of clashes they may encounter in their contact with certain types of patients.

Several studies have shown that some therapists do not like to treat low-income patients and, in fact, consider such treatment a waste of time (Lorion, 1973, 1974). Studies also indicate that even clinical supervisors tend to denigrate the merit of trying to find ways to help low-income patients.

Mental health systems are not alone in offering services that discriminate against the poor, the working-class, and the minority patient. In the area of general health care systems, low-income groups generally receive less physician care than more affluent groups, despite the evidence that medical need increases as one's income decreases (U.S. Department of Health, Education, and Welfare, 1979).

A number of studies have indicated that low-income, poorly educated patients are accepted less often into psychotherapy or into mental health services than are other types of individuals (Brill & Storrow, 1960; Hollingshead & Redlich, 1958; Rosenthal & Frank, 1958). Further, these patients typically continue for a shorter time or show higher dropout rates (Baekeland & Lundwall, 1975). The exact reasons for these phenomena are not known. Either patients are not requesting treatment, or they are disappointed with the kind of treatment they receive, or they resolve their problems more quickly and therefore leave therapy sooner than other patients. The underservicing of these individuals may also be a result of therapists selecting other patients who are similar to themselves in verbal fluency, economic level, and ethnic background (Yamamoto, James, Bloombaum, & Hattem, 1967). In summary, therapists may not be as readily accepting of poor, working-class, or minority patients into treatment or may be giving subtle messages to the patients that they are not interested in treating them.

Improper stereotyping of the poor by psychotherapists can lead to bias and error in diagnostic evaluation and psychotherapy (Goldstein, 1971). Misinformation or bias about a group's standards for normal and abnormal behavior may lead to error in diagnosis and judgment. Several investigators strongly suggest that bias can affect diagnosis and disposition, that is, the determination of which patients receive treatment and for how long (Karno, 1966; Lorion, 1973; Padilla, Ruiz, & Alvarez, 1975; Thomas & Sillen, 1972; Yamamoto *et al.*, 1967). Lorion (1974) has reviewed a number of studies in which experienced therapists, trainees, and supervisors have all expressed much discontent, frustration, and unwillingness to offer therapy to low-income patients. Much remains to be learned about error in diagnosis and treatment because of incorrect stereotypes about different cultural group norms and backgrounds (King, 1978).

The viewpoint that bias can affect therapy is not held by all mental health professionals. For example, some therapists argue that bias or prejudice is not allowed to affect the interaction with patients by trained, sensitive mental health professionals. With adequate training, diagnosis and treatment dispositions are strictly based on the objective findings about what is best for the patient. Proponents of this viewpoint suggest that acceptance or rejection of a patient into therapy is based on established and proven criteria. These criteria for acceptance to treatment include, for example, the patient's age, education, intelligence, social class, motivation, psychological-mindedness, insightfulness, and freedom from external constraints. Advocates of this viewpoint argue that these criteria may be applied without bias providing that the therapists are adequately trained.

Characteristics of Poor, Working-Class, and Minority Patients

Compared to more affluent patients, some differences do appear to exist in the life orientation of low-income patients, and these may interfere with traditional psychotherapy. They tend to be less obsessional about how they relate to life. Further, they live on such a limited economic plane that setbacks more easily become crises. They are thus much less likely to accept a plan of therapy which may take several months or even years. Rather, they may need and probably assume that resolutions to their psychological stress will be reached in the very near future. Effective therapy must match these expectations or attempt to change them.

In addition, there may be a lesser emphasis on verbalization and a greater emphasis on action for the low-income white, or minority patient. For example, a working-class patient may communicate the wish to discontinue therapy and then just stop attending without further discussion. A middle-class patient, on the other hand, may discuss this issue over the course of several interviews with the therapist.

Finally, the therapist must realize that there is a tendency to stereotype the working class, the poor, and minorities as being "losers" because they do not fit the stereotype the therapists have of "winners" who are like themselves. Poor people are easily considered blameworthy for being in that situation. Professionals often believe that everyone should side with the American success formula of individualism, hard work, and perseverance. Those who are not in a "success" level are then seen as "losers" in the races to riches, power, and status.

Characteristics of the Psychotherapist

The characteristics of psychotherapists can also interfere with effective psychotherapy. In fact, one recent study involving low-income Hispanic, black, and white outpatients found the reason most frequently given by these patients for prematurely terminating therapy was a negative reaction to the therapist (Acosta, 1980).

The social perspectives of the psychotherapist and the traditional model of a good patient may greatly hinder effective psychotherapy. The well-known YAVIS patient first described by Schofield (1964) is young, attractive, verbal, intelligent, and successful. The YAVIS patient is the one that most therapists naturally seek. For the most part, patients who come from the poor and the working classes and belong to minority groups do not fulfill the YAVIS stereotype. Such patients may be looking for relief from problems of living. Their objectives may be very limited and simple. If patients do not directly communicate these issues to the therapist, the therapist may make inappropriate inferences about their problems or requests.

Ignorance of the patient's life-style may lead the therapist to make assumptions that are incorrect and possibly disadvantageous to the patient. For example, a resident listened to a woman patient's complaints, thought he understood what the patient's problems were, and continued therapy with the patient based on his perception of her problems. One day he made a home visit to the patient under the auspices of a community psychiatry class assignment. This visit was indeed an eye-opener for the resident. He found that the patient, her husband, and several children were living in a tiny, run-down apartment under severely deprived circumstances. The witnessing of these very real problems caused him to change the focus of treatment from merely talking with the patient, to actively trying to help her and her family cope with their social reality. Happily, the resident's efforts in dealing with the patient's reality problems were successful, and the patient was able to move into a more appropriate apartment without the cramped conditions and difficulties of the previous apartment. This lessening of the patient's preoccupation with her reality problems in turn enabled the talking therapy to proceed more effectively.

Related to the above example is the message that therapists may often be unwilling to accept the dual nature, the "double neediness," of the therapy that is often required by the poor because of their frequently deprived circumstances. This combination therapy is a mixture of psychotherapy plus psychosocial therapy. The psychotherapy component often may be time limited, supportive, and direct. The psychosocial therapy component involves an understanding of the social circumstances of the patient, together with appropriate and active interventions when indicated.

For example, during an initial evaluation with a middle-aged black woman, she insisted that she needed only a minor tranquilizer, which she had "always" received from doctors for the past twenty years. With sensitive questioning, the therapist learned of the woman's increased anxiety and depression because of the loss of work resulting from illness and her inability to get straight answers from the welfare office, physicians, the Social Security office, and attorneys. Her biggest stress was caused by her inability to pay her bills. Her life history revealed that she had always worked, sometimes holding two jobs simultaneously, since she was 8 years old. She was also suffering from the toll on her family of ghetto-life stress—several family members were very ill, one son was dead, and one son was recuperating from a violent assault and unable to find work. The therapist created a short-term contract with her to see him four times. He also introduced her to a clinic caseworker to intervene directly and immediately with the public agencies, which were bogged down in red tape. The patient was pleased with this quick action and volunteered that maybe after the fourth session she could talk about her feelings and learn to become happier in her life.

The problem, as we conceptualize it, lies in the dyad, the patient–therapist relationship, and not simply in the patient as a bad patient. The working-class, the poor, and the minorities in general have meager educational backgrounds which makes it difficult for the well-educated middle-class mental health professional to understand and communicate with the patient. The effect of these different experiences and life styles must be understood and accepted by the therapist in order to improve therapy for the poor and minorities.

Now please complete the Self-Assessment Exercise 1.1.

SELF-ASSESSMENT EXERCISE 1.1

1. Describe what is meant by "double neediness."

2. What is meant by a YAVIS patient?

3. On the scales below indicate the position that best describes the poor, the working-class, the low-income white, and the minority patient.

a. High verbal fluency	└─┴─┴─┴─┘	Low verbal fluency
b. High income level	└─┴─┴─┴─┘	Low income level
c. Adequate resources to handle problems of living	└─┴─┴─┴─┘	Inadequate resources to handle problems of living
d. High educational level	└─┴─┴─┴─┘	Low educational level
e. Low unemployment level	└─┴─┴─┴─┘	High unemployment level
f. "Winners" attitude	└─┴─┴─┴─┘	"Losers" attitude
g. Believes destiny is under personal control	└─┴─┴─┴─┘	Believes destiny is controlled by outside forces
h. Uses English language exclusively	└─┴─┴─┴─┘	Uses foreign language or ethnic dialect exclusively

9

4. On the scales below indicate the position that best describes the therapist in a typical mental health facility.

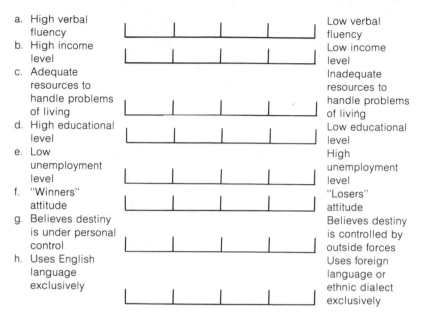

a. High verbal fluency	Low verbal fluency
b. High income level	Low income level
c. Adequate resources to handle problems of living	Inadequate resources to handle problems of living
d. High educational level	Low educational level
e. Low unemployment level	High unemployment level
f. "Winners" attitude	"Losers" attitude
g. Believes destiny is under personal control	Believes destiny is controlled by outside forces
h. Uses English language exclusively	Uses foreign language or ethnic dialect exclusively

5. Describe the potential effects on each other and on the therapeutic outcome of the different characteristics of patients and therapists.

When you complete this exercise, check your answers with those that follow.

SELF-ASSESSMENT EXERCISE 1.1: FEEDBACK

1. "Double neediness" means that in addition to having emotional problems, some patients also have reality-based problems of living that they are unable to handle.

2. A YAVIS patient is young, attractive, verbal, intelligent, and successful. Therapists seem to choose these patients for treatment because they can more clearly identify with them and their problems.

3. The poor, the working class, the low-income white, and the minority patient would be described in the following way:

a. High verbal fluency	`|___|___|_X_|___|___|`	Low verbal fluency
b. High income level	`|___|___|___|_X_|___|`	Low income level
c. Adequate resources to handle problems of living	`|___|___|___|_X_|___|`	Inadequate resources to handle problems of living
d. High educational level	`|___|___|___|_X_|___|`	Low educational level
e. Low unemployment level	`|___|___|___|_X_|___|`	High unemployment level
f. "Winners" attitude	`|___|___|_X_|___|___|`	"Losers" attitude
g. Believes destiny is under personal control	`|___|___|_X_|___|___|`	Believes destiny is controlled by outside forces
h. Uses English language exclusively	`|___|___|_X_|___|___|`	Uses foreign language or ethnic dialect exclusively

4. The therapist would be described in the following way:

a. High verbal fluency	`|_X_|___|___|___|___|`	Low verbal fluency
b. High income level	`|_X_|___|___|___|___|`	Low income level
c. Adequate resources to handle problems of living	`|_X_|___|___|___|___|`	Inadequate resources to handle problems of living

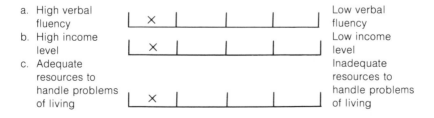

11

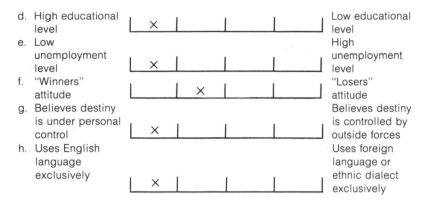

d. High educational level / Low educational level
e. Low unemployment level / High unemployment level
f. "Winners" attitude / "Losers" attitude
g. Believes destiny is under personal control / Believes destiny is controlled by outside forces
h. Uses English language exclusively / Uses foreign language or ethnic dialect exclusively

5. There is much debate about the effect on the therapeutic outcome, if any, of differences between the characteristics of the typical patient and the typical therapist. Some effects may be: greater difficulty in obtaining service, shorter service, inaccurate diagnoses, ineffective disposition (treatment), and lack of interest in treating the patient. Therapists feel they can't help the patient; the patient feels therapists don't care to help.

If your answers correspond closely with those above, continue your reading. Otherwise reread the preceding material.

PATIENT REQUESTS FOR PSYCHIATRIC SERVICES

Poor, working-class, and minority people come to a mental health outpatient clinic for a variety of reasons; however, current research indicates that there seems to be little inter-social class difference in what people expect of therapists and treatment (Lorion, 1973). Although the reasons are many, some investigators have managed to effectively identify specific categories or clusters of reasons. For example, Lazare, Eisenthal, Wasserman, and Harford (1975) at the Massachusetts General Hospital have categorized the requests of over 600 low-income and minority patients during several years of careful research. The following 15 categories were derived from black and white patients of both sexes who were being seen for the first time in an adult psychiatric walk-in clinic (each category will show patient statements as examples).

Administrative Request. Request for help in dealing with bureaucracy, agencies, and so forth. For example: "I need the clinic's authority to deal with a certain agency I am having trouble with." "I need the clinic's legal power to take care of a difficult situation for me."

Advice. Request for specific guidance on personal to nonpersonal matters. For example: "If someone could tell me the right thing to do about my personal affairs, I would be helped." "I thought you might know better than I what I ought to do about a problem in my life now (job, where to live, finances, etc.)."

Clarification. Request for help in putting feelings, thoughts, or behavior in some perspective. For example: "I want to clarify how I feel about certain things." "I want to clear things up to make the best decision for myself."

Community Triage. Request for information on where in the community to get needed services. For example: "I would like someone to tell me where in my community I can get help." "I would like you to direct me to the agency in my community which can help me with my problems."

Confession. Request to talk to the therapist and ease guilt feelings arising out of something the patient said, thought, or did. For example: "I want to confess to someone what I have thought or done." "I feel like I need to be forgiven."

Control. The patient feels overwhelmed and out of control and is requesting the therapist to take over and take control of the patient's life. For example: "Keep me from falling apart." "I'm losing my mind. I need help."

Set Limits. Requests for the clinician to protect the patient by setting firm and consistent limits. For example: "I want someone who can say no to me." "I want someone who will not let me get away with things."

Nothing. These patients have no requests. For example: "Someone else brought me here, but I do not need psychiatric care." "I was sent here by the other clinic and don't know why I'm here."

Medical. Requests for medical treatment to "cure" the patient. For example: "I want someone to examine me to figure out the cause of my nervous condition." "I'm nervous and can't sleep. I'd like to get something to calm me down."

Psychodynamic Insight. The patient wants to talk about problems which are perceived by the patient as originating in his or her early development. For example: "I think a lot of my problems are related to my past. I'd like to talk to someone so I can learn to overcome them." "I want to talk about my childhood, where all my problems began."

Psychological Expertise. The patient wants an explanation as to why he or she thinks, feels, or acts in a particular way. For example: "I want someone to tell me why I do the things I do." "If someone could explain to me what causes my emotional problems, I would be helped."

Reality Contact. Request for the clinician to help the patient "check out" or "keep in touch with" reality so that the patient won't feel he or she is "going crazy." For example: "I want to talk to someone so I will feel sane." "I have to find out if what just happened to me is real."

Social Intervention. Requests for the clinic to use its social influence and intervene on the patient's behalf to alleviate problems which the patient perceives as residing primarily in other people or situations. For example: "My problem is someone else (family, friends, or at work). I want you to do something about them." "I want you to speak to the person or people who are giving me trouble."

Succorance. Requests for a person to be warm, caring, involved, and comforting to the patient. For example: "I'm here because I need the warmth of human contact." "I would like someone to help me feel less lonely and empty."

Ventilation. Request to tell the clinician various feelings (not guilt-laden, as in confession) in an effort to feel better by getting them out in the open. For example: "I want to express my angry feelings." "I want to get some painful feelings out of my system."

"ACCEPTABLE" AND "UNACCEPTABLE" REQUESTS

These request categories may be loosely divided into those anticipated and accepted as genuine therapeutic activities by most psychotherapists and those which may be misunderstood or rejected by some psychotherapists. Among those that are usually *accepted* are Advice, Clarification, Confession, Control, Limits, Psychodynamic Insight, Psychological Expertise, Reality Contact, Succorance, and Ventilation. Note that the requests accepted by therapists as legitimate reasons for coming to an outpatient mental health clinic generally deal with the treatment of emotional problems.

The types of requests that may be misunderstood or *not accepted* by therapists are: Administrative Request, Community Triage, Nothing, Medical, and Social Intervention. These misunderstood reasons generally relate to a patient's problems of living but are in fact legitimate areas for a therapist to deal with.

The following paragraphs present brief discussions of each category of patient request not commonly accepted by therapists and illustrate some of the possible ways therapists can help patients deal with their problems of living.

Administrative Requests. Patients come to the clinic with problems which may require constructive administrative action on the therapist's part. For example, the following patient–therapist dialogue may take place:

PATIENT: I need the clinic's help because I got busted for drunk driving.
THERAPIST: I'm not sure what I can do about that; I'm not an attorney.
PATIENT: I'm afraid they might put me in jail or worse yet, put me in
    jail and take away my driver's license.

Here, the therapist should be aware that police more frequently patrol areas where minorities and poor people live and that arrests for drunk driving are consequently higher than in other areas (Morales, 1972, chap. 4). This is an example of an important reality problem which the patient has and with which you may help him, even though you are not an attorney. You may wish to assess both the patient's overall drinking behavior (for example, is alcoholism part of the problem or not) and the immediate problem. If appropriate, you may then send a report to the judge that is supportive of your patient's ability to continue to function in the community. The legal system will often positively consider supportive information from mental health professionals.

A different example of an administrative request may be a situation that calls on you to prepare a statement concerning the inability of your patient to work for psychological reasons. This request often poses a problem for middle-class therapists because of their own work ethic. If the patient looks physically healthy, there is often a strong reluctance to write a statement indicating that the patient is justified to miss work "simply" for psychological reasons. It is important that therapists not allow their own biases and preferences to interfere with an appropriate and accurate clinical judgment.

Community Triage. A patient may say, "I'd like someone to tell me where in my community to get help." Then she might reveal a specific problem, for example, being beaten by her husband, which has resulted in not only physical harm, but increasing anxiety with symptoms reflective of the trauma. This patient would need not only psychotherapy to reassure and ease the level of anxiety, but also advice about shelters where she might be protected and where she can get information about how best to cope with this difficult marital situation.

Another patient may be having a problem with her husband who is a chronic alcohol abuser. The patient may complain of the serious drunkenness of her husband and the fact that he's out of work now. The family is suffering not only the deleterious effects of his alcoholism but financial deprivation as well. As the therapist, you may suggest a detoxification center for the husband, together with a referral to Alcoholics Anonymous. The wife could then be seen for a few more times to make sure that appropriate help has been obtained and that she is feeling better. Another alternative might be to suggest conjoint therapy to help the husband and wife deal with his alcohol abuse.

Nothing. It is important to note that among the low-income patients, only a very small percentage will be self-referred to a mental health outpatient facility (Acosta, 1980). Many reasons may account for this, ranging from basic lack of familiarity with mental health treatment systems to social taboos. What is even more troublesome, however, is that many patients will be referred by a social agency, a physician, a medical clinic, a friend, or a relative without the benefit of any discussion, exploration, or explanation to account for the referral. The result, then, is that patients may legitimately arrive at a mental health facility and tell a therapist that they have *nothing* to request.

On occasions when an individual has no request, therapists must become educators to these patients and take a few minutes to explain who they are and how they can be of service to people. It is important for a naive patient to know what specific services are available to him or her, as in the following example:

THERAPIST: How can I help you?
PATIENT: I don't know, man. You tell me. I see this place is a psychiatric

clinic. I'm not crazy or mentally disturbed. I don't know why I'm even here.

THERAPIST: Well, why do you think?

PATIENT: Like I say, I don't know. All I know is that I'm following my doctor's orders. You know, he told me to come over here and even made me this appointment with you.

THERAPIST: Your doctor didn't explain to you why he thought you should see someone here?

PATIENT: No.

THERAPIST: I see. Let me explain who I am and what I do. Maybe then we can talk some more and figure out why your doctor thought I could help you.

In the above example we can see that if a therapist does not take the time or interest to help the patient become oriented to the service, the patient can easily be lost to any mental health intervention that is needed. On the other hand, when a patient presents with "nothing," it is critical to insure an evaluation or intervention actually is needed. Sometimes the person who called in to schedule the patient's appointment contacted the wrong facility.

Medical Requests. A patient may ask to be examined physically because of being very nervous and having tremendous insomnia and agitation. The therapist can talk to the patient in terms of the request for medical help and point out that these symptoms may be related to psychological distress. The therapist should then assess the need for an examination and, if that need exists, recommend a physical examination. However, continued evaluation and psychological help should be provided.

Social Intervention. A young mother may say, "I have a problem with my son who wets his bed every night. Please tell me what I could do about this." As the therapist, you could either advise about the various ways in which enuresis is treated if you are knowledgeable, or you could make an appointment for the patient with a child therapist. Often patients come to us because they have little in the way of social support systems, including individuals to advise them about unique human problems.

As another example the patient may say, "I'd like to have you speak to my employer because I felt too sick to work. The employer is complaining about my being on sick leave all the time." You could evaluate the extent of the time taken off for sick leave, the patient's psychological condition, its relationship to your treatment, and advice that would be appropriate.

All these requests should be carefully considered by therapists, who should then take an action which they feel is appropriate. Sometimes this action will support the patient's request and sometimes it will not. However, in every case the patient should know that the request was important enough to have received the therapist's careful consideration.

Now please complete the Self-Assessment Exercise 1.2.

SELF-ASSESSMENT EXERCISE 1.2

1. List each of the patient reasons for coming to a mental health clinic which are generally anticipated and accepted by therapists.

2. Describe the general theme which underlies all of these reasons.

3. List each of the patient reasons for coming to a mental health clinic which are generally not anticipated and accepted by therapists.

4. Describe the general theme which underlies all of these reasons.

When you complete the exercise, please check your answers with those that follow.

SELF-ASSESSMENT EXERCISE 1.2: FEEDBACK

1. Accepted reasons are: advice, clarification, confession, control, insight, set limits, psychological expertise, reality contact, succorance, and ventilation.

2. They all deal with the treatment of emotional problems.

3. Reasons which are not generally accepted are: administrative request, community triage, nothing, medical, and social intervention.

4. These reasons generally deal with problems of living and do not have a precipitating emotional cause.

If your answers correspond closely with those above, please continue your reading. Otherwise, reread the previous material.

TREATMENT ISSUES

Specific Patient–Therapist Interaction

Typical Communication Problem. Poor, working-class, low-income white or minority patients may often show reluctance to express or disclose their deep feelings, attitudes, problems, and requests. We have observed this phenomena over a number of years of clinical practice and training of therapists. The psychiatric and psychological literature is replete with reports of therapists' frustration with poor patients who are not highly verbal and disclosing (Lorion, 1973, 1974). Patients may easily see the therapist as a powerful authority figure and feel highly distanced. Patients may then be afraid to tell the middle-class therapist what they want directly, if they disagree, or if there are problems related to their actual treatment. For example, patients are often reluctant to discuss their difficulties or disagreements with the therapist's plans for treatment duration. In other words, they fail to assert themselves. This is not a surprising phenomenon. Consider, for example, that the general American public has evolved a high level of respect for medical doctors, to the point of often seeing them as god-like. This attitude affects both rich and poor. It has more suppressing effects, however, on the people who cannot match the educational and economic prowess of doctors. Typically, individuals with firmer economic foundations are more prone to question and challenge authority, since they feel more entitled to customer satisfaction.

Patient Assertive Statements. It is important to try to change the patients' behavior so that they will speak more directly and openly. Therapists can encourage *more assertive* communication as well as reinforce these statements by actively listening to patients "telling it like it is" and by responding in a positive manner. Therapists must then take whatever actions are appropriate to solve the problems being expressed.

Patient assertive statements are statements or questions to the therapist, stating an opinion or preference, expressing plans or change of plans, clarifying the patient's position or viewpoint, clarifying the patient–therapist relationship, or stating a disagreement between the patient and therapist. Assertive statements must directly relate to and involve the therapist. In short, assertive statements are expressions of a person's human right to agree or disagree, in an appropriate manner, with someone else. When an individual disagrees with another in an inappropriate manner, for example, at the expense of the other person's own rights, feelings, or self-esteem, the disagreeing behavior could be termed aggressive behavior and should not be encouraged.

As an illustration, suppose a patient agrees to return for an 8:00 A.M. appointment in one week when he doesn't really want to keep the appointment. He is behaving passively at the moment. The chances are high that he won't keep the appointment! On the other hand, if the patient stated that he really didn't like the 8:00 A.M. appointment and would like a later time, he would be acting assertively. The appointment time may or may not be changed, but at least the patient would have spoken up and given the therapist an opportunity to find a better time and to learn of the patient's disagreement.

Additionally, assertive statements may directly seek the therapist's help with some problem of living, for example, "Could you please write a note to my boss asking permission for me to leave work early to come to the clinic?"

Patient Aggressive Statements. Aggressive statements are to be distinguished from assertive statements. Aggressive statements are those which express a person's wishes, but at the expense of another person. For example, aggressive statements would include those which are threatening, insulting, obscene, or menacing. Aggressive statements, while often revealing topics which are emotionally charged for the patient, are generally not conducive to productive therapy.

Patient Self-Disclosure Statements. Therapists should also encourage self-disclosure statements by the patient. This encouragement will facilitate more efficient therapy. These are statements made by a patient that convey personal information. This information is generally private and would not normally be shared with a stranger. It may involve attitudes, behaviors, thoughts, emotions, or problems. These strictly personal statements may also relate to a patient's feelings about the therapist, for example, "I often feel sad," or "I get extremely nervous when I'm in an elevator all by myself," or "I find it hard to talk to you."

General Therapeutic Recommendations. Many of the patients who come to a public mental health outpatient clinic are not suitable for insight-oriented therapy alone. These patients actually require a mixture of therapies to meet their double neediness. The patients' emotional problems should be considered co-equal with their problems of living. This requires the mental health professional to be viewed not only as a psychotherapist but at times as an adviser or an advocate who helps patients deal with individuals and agencies involved in their problems of living. Such comprehensive therapy requires that therapists become familiar with the real-life situation of their patients. In addition, therapists must become aware of and utilize the available paraprofessional staff, for example, medical case workers, community workers, or community aides, who have been trained to help therapists deal with patients' multiple problems of living.

A second recommendation is that therapy should be conceptualized into time-limited segments of perhaps six or fewer visits at a time. This helps to maintain specific short-range goals toward which both patient and therapist can work. At the end of each period, a new treatment segment should then be renegotiated. Therapeutic objectives must be clear and acceptable to both patient and therapist.

A third recommendation is that if the therapist begins to experience prejudicial attitudes toward the patient arising from the patient's minority or low-income status, the therapist must deal directly with them. Active, supportive consultation with another mental health professional would be beneficial for the therapist to help alleviate prejudice. Such consultations should preferably be with individuals who are particularly concerned and experienced with the problems of the poor, working-class, and minority patients.

It must be remembered that despite these generalizations, treatment must be tailored to the individual needs of each patient. Regardless of a patient's socioeconomic or ethnic background, flexible, individualized therapy is a necessity.

Now please complete the Self-Assessment Exercise 1.3.

SELF-ASSESSMENT EXERCISE 1.3

1. Describe the typical communication problem which low-income and minority patients often encounter with therapists.

2. Describe what therapists can do to change low-income and minority patient communication problems.

3. Describe assertive statements.

4. Describe self-disclosure statements.

5. Distinguish between assertive and aggressive statements.

6. Describe four general therapeutic recommendations which were discussed.

When you have completed this exercise, check your answers with those that follow.

SELF-ASSESSMENT EXERCISE 1.3: FEEDBACK

1. The typical patient–therapist communication problem is one in which the patient regards the therapist as an authority figure and is reluctant to express deep feelings, problems, or disagreements with the therapists.

2. Therapists should encourage their patients to be more open and direct by showing interest in their statements. They should encourage open and direct communication and reinforce it when it occurs. They should take actions to solve as many of the patient's problems as possible. *also modeling/suggesting*

3. A patient assertive statement is a statement or question by the patient to the therapist stating an opinion or preference, expressing plans or change of plans, clarifying the patient's position or viewpoint, clarifying the patient–therapist relationship, or stating a disagreement between the patient and therapist. Assertive statements must directly relate to and involve the therapist.

4. A patient self-disclosure statement is a statement made by a patient which conveys personal information. This information is generally private and would not normally be shared with a stranger. It may involve attitudes, behaviors, thoughts, emotions, or problems. These statements by the patient are strictly personal and may also relate to the patient's feelings about the therapist.

5. Aggressive statements are those which express a person's wishes but at the expense of another person. They may be threatening, insulting, obscene, or menacing.

6. Therapeutic recommendations include the following:

   a. Be prepared to deal with the double neediness of your patients.
   b. Conceptualize therapy into short time-limited segments.
   c. Obtain help in overcoming any prejudices you discover in yourself.
   d. Provide flexible, individualized therapy.

If your answers are similar to those above, continue your reading. Otherwise, please reread the preceding sections.

SUMMARY

The vast majority of Americans belong to the working classes and poor. Hollingshead's (1957) *Two-Factor Index of Social Position* es-

timates that perhaps 70% of Americans belong to Class IV (low-income, working class) and Class V (poor, unemployed, unskilled).
Recent estimates indicate that this percentage has not substantially
changed (Hauge, 1972). This being the case, we hope that the preceding material will help you work more effectively with most
Americans.

Insight therapy is appropriate only with a small and select group
of Americans. Many people visting mental health outpatient clinics
want brief treatment and practical coping help. In these instances,
our patients are our customers. As such we hope that they will be
met with courtesy, be treated with respect, and that their requests,
wishes, and needs will be listened to with understanding. When it
is possible to meet these requests within the limits of our therapeutic
capabilities, we believe that it is appropriate to do so. If it is not
possible to fulfill the patient's request, you should explain why it
isn't. Although a patient may be frustrated and disappointed, it is
better for a patient to have a clear explanation of what is possible in
the context of a mental health facility than to labor under a false
expectation.

REFERENCES

Acosta, F. X. Ethnic variables in psychotherapy: The Mexican American. In J. L. Mar-
    tinez (Ed.), Chicano psychology. New York: Academic Press, 1977.
Acosta, F. X. Self-described reasons for premature termination of psychotherapy by
    Mexican American, Black American, and Anglo-American patients. Psychological
    Reports, 1980, 47, 435–443.
Baekeland, F., & Lundwall, L. Dropping out of treatment: A critical review. Psychological
    Bulletin, 1975, 82, 738–783.
Brill, N. Q., & Storrow, H. A. Social class and psychiatric treatment. Archives of General
    Psychiatry, 1960, 3, 340–344.
Goldstein, A. P. Psychotherapeutic attraction. New York: Pergamon, 1971.
Hauge, M. Social class measurement; Methodological critique. In G. W. Thielbar & S.
    B. Feldman (Eds.), Issues in social inequality. Boston: Little, Brown, 1972.
Hollingshead, A. B. Two-factor index of social position. Unpublished manuscript, Yale
    University, 1957.
Hollingshead, A. B., & Redlich, F. C. Social class and mental illness: A community study.
    New York: Wiley, 1958.
Karno, M. The enigma of ethnicity in a psychiatric clinic. Archives of General Psychiatry,
    1966, 14, 516–520.
King, L. M. Social and cultural influences on psychopathology. Annual Review of Psy-
    chology, 1978, 29, 405–433.

Lazare, A., Eisenthal, S., Wasserman, L., & Harford, T. Patient requests in a walk-in clinic. *Comprehensive Psychiatry*, 1975, *16*, 467–477.

Lorion, R. P. Socioeconomic status and traditional treatment approaches reconsidered. *Psychological Bulletin*, 1973, *79*, 263–270.

Lorion, R. P. Patient and therapist variables in the treatment of low-income patients. *Psychological Bulletin*, 1974, *81*, 344–354.

Morales, A. *Ando sangrando (I am bleeding): A study of Mexican American–police conflict.* La Puente, Calif.: Perspectiva Publications, 1972.

Padilla, A. M., Ruiz, R. A., & Alvarez, R. Community mental health services for the Spanish-speaking/surnamed population. *American Psychologist*, 1975, *30*, 892–905.

President's Commission on Mental Health. *Report to the President* (Vol. 1). Washington, D.C.: U.S. Government Printing Office, 1978.

Rosenthal, D., & Frank, J. D. The fate of psychiatric clinic outpatients assigned to psychotherapy. *Journal of Nervous and Mental Disease*, 1958, *127*, 330–343.

Schofield, W. *Psychotherapy: The purchase of friendship.* Englewood Cliffs, N.J.: Prentice-Hall, 1964.

Sue, S. Community mental health services to minority groups: Some optimism, some pessimism. *American Psychologist*, 1977, *32*, 616–624.

Thomas, A., & Sillen, S. *Racism and psychiatry.* New York: Brunner/Mazel, 1972.

U.S. Department of Health, Education, and Welfare. *Health status of minorities and low-income groups* (Public Health Service, Health Resources Opportunity Publication No. HRA 79-627). Washington, D.C.: U.S. Government Printing Office, 1979.

Yamamoto, J., James, Q. C., Bloombaum, M., & Hattem, J. Racial factors in patient selection. *American Journal of Psychiatry*, 1967, *124*, 630–636.

Yamamoto, J., James, Q. C., & Palley, N. Cultural problems in psychiatric therapy. *Archives of General Psychiatry*, 1968, *19*, 45–49.

CHAPTER 2

The Poor and Working-Class Patient

Joe Yamamoto, Frank X. Acosta, and Leonard A. Evans

INTRODUCTION

A significant part of our population in the United States are people
who fall into the poor or working-class categories (Hollingshead &
Redlich, 1958; U.S. Bureau of Census, 1974). An even higher percentage of patients coming to public psychiatric outpatient clinics or
community mental health centers fall into these categories. The National Institute of Mental Health (NIMH) has increasingly recognized
in the past several years the need to augment services for these groups
of people. Typically, the poor and the working class are not being
helped effectively in mental health services, even though such clinics
and centers have been created for them (President's Commission on
Mental Health, 1978). In realization of these conditions, NIMH has
in the past few years moved toward the idea of educating the general
medical practitioner to be the primary provider of mental health services for the low-income person.

The poor and working classes are defined by the level of education attained and the occupation of the primary wage earners (Coleman & Rainwater, 1978; Hollingshead & Redlich, 1958). The purpose
of this chapter is to describe the characteristics of members of these
classes and to provide advice for the therapist who is treating a member of this group.

After completing this chapter and a corresponding group discussion session, the reader should be able to:

1. Describe the characteristics of poor and working-class patients
2. Describe the important attitudes of poor and working-class
   patients regarding psychotherapy

3. Describe the problems commonly faced by therapists in treating such patients
4. Describe and use therapeutic approaches and actions which are most effective with this clientele
5. Express satisfaction with the process and outcome of therapeutic encounters with poor and working-class patients

Please read these learning objectives until you become familiar with the goals of this chapter, then begin reading the following section.

CHARACTERISTICS OF POOR AND WORKING-CLASS PATIENTS

Two decades ago, Hollingshead and Redlich (1958) published their pioneering book *Social Class and Mental Illness*. These investigators carefully documented and described diverse and unequal treatment of patients in both outpatient and inpatient settings, depending on the patient's social class. Essentially, poor and working-class patients were receiving briefer forms of therapy and more chemotherapy than were middle- and upper-class patients. Indeed, even the incidence of mental illness was found to be higher among the poor. Diagnostic practices were such that the poor were more often labeled as being severely mentally disordered, while the rich were labeled as being mildly to moderately distressed.

Hollingshead and Redlich's work was important not only for its creative and revealing aspects but also for its scientific approach in defining social class. Using education and occupation as criteria, Hollingshead and Redlich divided Americans into five classes. They showed that the five social classes had unequal distribution, that is, there was not a 20% distribution in Class I, II, III, IV, and V, respectively. Table 2.1 shows the actual distributions. It is important to realize that a large proportion of Americans still fall into the working class (Class IV) and the poor class (Class V) (Redlich & Kellert, 1978; U.S. Bureau of Census, 1974).

The working class is sometimes referred to as the blue-collar class. Even though blue-collar workers may actually earn more money than some white-collar workers who comprise the middle, or some of the upper middle class, their life-styles differ significantly.

Table 2.1. Distribution of Social Class in the
United States

Social class	%
I Upper class	3.4
II Upper middle class	9.0
III Middle class	21.4
IV Lower middle class (working class)	48.5
V Lower class (poor)	17.7

The working class is part of the American mainstream. As such, they have jobs and many American advantages such as television, automobiles, and so forth. Although inflation in recent years has robbed them of many of the additional benefits of the working-class life-style, they have not despaired of the American Dream. For example, their expressed desires about what they want for themselves in psychotherapy (Frank, Eisenthal, & Lazare, 1978) and also for their children in education and life are quite similar to the aspirations of the middle class and the upper middle class, but their life-style in terms of education, experience, and work is at a different level (Hill, 1971). They have not achieved the American middle-class dream of education and occupational advancement. Therefore, they have settled for a life-style of working in their regular jobs and have maintained the dream in terms of recreational interests and verbalized aspirations.

In their classical work, Hollingshead and Redlich (1958) summarized the working class family life:

> They now live in a two-family home, are satisfied with their housing, but hope to buy a single family home in the suburbs some day. They have four or five children; the younger ones are in elementary and high school; the oldest one has finished school and is working on the production line of a local factory or, if male, is in the Armed Services. The husband and father has been working since the age of seventeen. He worked at his first job for about a year and a half, then changed to one that he thought was better; however, he is still a semi-skilled worker on a production line. His wife, too, began to work in the factory when she was seventeen years of age, but she may have tried sales or clerical jobs as well. She worked at her first job for about two years. She was working when she was married and continued to work until her first pregnancy was well advanced.
>
> The recreation of the parents consists of working around the place, viewing television, occasionally listening to the radio, some reading and family visiting. The children spend more time with television, radio, and

the movies than do their parents. In addition, they go to local athletic events and visit the amusement park two or three times during the season. The husband belongs to the "Union" but not other organizations. The wife belongs to no formal organizations, but is a member of an informal neighborhood women's group. The effective family income in this description is limited and savings may have to be used to pay for emergencies. Although the family may feel economically secure they are not wholly satisfied with their living conditions and the children are dissatisfied. (p. 113)

People in Class IV, the working class, tend to belong to unions, to be skilled or semiskilled, to have regular employment, to have a high school education and diploma, and to show relatively more family instability than higher social-class groups (Hollingshead & Redlich, 1958).

On the other hand, people in Class V, the poor class, tend to be nonunion members, to be more unskilled, to have more irregular employment, and more unemployment, to have less than a high school education, and to show more degree of family instability than Class IV.

There are important distinctions for therapists to be aware of in working with patients from either Class IV or Class V. For example, Class IV persons have more opportunity to achieve middle-class possessions and goals. However, both classes are usually unable to participate in the race for prestige and status enjoyed by the upper-class and upper-middle-class groups.

Interestingly, people in Class V, the poor class, are those who receive the most discrimination. Even members of Class IV discriminate and are prejudiced against members from Class V. How much more could this be true for members of upper classes?

Several authors, for example, Allen (1970), Fishman (1969), and Thomas and Sillen (1972) have noted that there is little solid empirical information available about the feelings, aspirations, and behavior of the poor. As a result, there is much generalization and theorizing concerning members of these groups.

The objective information shown by several studies such as Dohrenwend and Dohrenwend (1974); Hollingshead and Redlich (1958); Srole, Langer, Michael, Opler, and Rennie (1962), do indicate that members of poor and working-class groups tend to show greater psychological distress and disorders than do other social classes.

Now please complete the Self-Assessment Exercise 2.1.

SELF-ASSESSMENT EXERCISE 2.1

1. Approximately 70% of Americans fall into social class _____ .

    a. III
    b. IV
    c. V
    d. III and II
    e. IV and V

2. Working-class individuals' expectations for themselves in psychotherapy and for their children in education are _____ the aspirations of middle- and upper-middle-class individuals.

    a. less than
    b. similar to
    c. greater than
    d. not comparable to
    e. identical to

3. Educational levels of middle-class white-collar workers compared to working-class blue-collar workers are _____ .

    a. greater
    b. similar
    c. less
    d. not discussed in text

4. Compare Class IV to Class V for the following characteristics:

	Class IV	Class V
a. More education	_____	_____
b. Union membership	_____	_____
c. Unskilled work	_____	_____
d. More family instability	_____	_____
e. More discrimination	_____	_____

When you have completed this exercise, check your answers with those that follow.

SELF-ASSESSMENT EXERCISE 2.1: FEEDBACK

1. A majority of Americans fall into social classes _____ .

   a. III
   b. IV
   c. V
   d. III and II
   (e.) IV and V

2. Working-class individuals' expectations for themselves in psychotherapy and for their children in education are _____ the aspirations of middle- and upper-middle-class individuals.

   a. less than
   (b.) similar to
   c. greater than
   d. not comparable to
   e. identical to

3. Educational levels of middle-class white-collar workers compared to working-class blue-collar workers are _____ .

   (a.) greater
   b. similar
   c. less
   d. not discussed in text

4. Compare Class IV to Class V for the following characteristics:

	Class IV	Class V
a. More education	X	
b. Union membership	X	
c. Unskilled work		X
d. More family instability		X
e. More discrimination		X

If your answers correspond closely with those above, please continue reading. If not, please reread the preceding material.

ATTITUDES TOWARD MENTAL HEALTH SERVICES

It is important to understand the life-styles and experiences of the working class. Gould (1967) has emphasized the importance of this understanding in his paper "Dr. Strangeclass." He described his efforts in working with these patients, whom he found to be quite different from those seen in his day-to-day private practice. In addition, evidence from the hospital insurance plan in New York suggested that the utilization of psychiatric services by the working class was quite different from that of the upper-middle-class professionals and middle-class professionals. The working class tend to need more encouragement to use mental health services appropriately and adequately. Without appropriate information and education, they tend to shy away from mental health services and seek the help of medical practitioners and other advisers instead.

Indeed, when Dr. Philip Wagner, a psychoanalyst prominent in Southern California, began his work as director of the mental health clinic for the Retail Clerks Union, he found that clinic services were unused. He began to inform members of the union about the services offered and the advantages of appropriate use of mental health help. Despite this, utilization was low until later, when the range of services offered was diversified from the usual mental health disciplines of psychiatry, psychology, and social work to include educational counselors, rehabilitation counselors, and many other helpers. These additions offered not only therapeutic and remedial services but educational and preventive work as well.

Among the working class there is a difference in the utilization patterns between men and women. This is not true for men and women who are professionals. Both male and female professionals tend to use mental health services equally. Among the working class, the women tend to use the services slightly more frequently. This may be in part a function of the availability of the services primarily during the day, when the working-class man may find it inconvenient to see a mental health worker. It is not known if such a difference holds up in clinics that offer therapy in the evening hours. Be that as it may, it is apparent that the utilization pattern differs for the sexes depending on the social class.

It was once believed that poor and working-class patients held primarily negative attitudes toward psychiatric treatment and that these patients were not interested in talking about their problems at any length to a professional, no matter how interested and willing to listen. More recently, studies have shown that there is little clear distinction among at least Classes III, IV, and V in their attitudes toward psychotherapy and in the kind of therapy which they seek.

For example, Lorion (1972) found in a clinic study that most patients across Classes III, IV, and V held positive attitudes toward therapy and were primarily interested in a therapist who was willing to listen. They were expecting to discuss personal and emotional issues with the therapist. These findings strongly suggest that even patients who are not well educated, who lack economic stability, and who have no general experience with therapists nonetheless have positive attitudes toward therapy and, if presented with the need and the opportunity, are interested in talking about their problems.

Unfortunately, such patients are more accustomed to seeing physicians rather than psychotherapists for problems that have an emotional basis. The conditioning and the role expectations developed from dialogue with physicians often interfere with effective interpersonal communication with a psychotherapist. Typically, for example, patients expect and receive very brief sessions with physicians, ranging from a few minutes to fifteen minutes. Typically, the physician asks a series of questions and the patient supplies the information. There tends to be little open-ended dialogue.

There is another important point to be made. Most poor and working-class people want the same things as other Americans, namely, the American Dream. This includes education, a decent job, suitable housing, and treatment with respect and consideration in one's day-to-day activities. However, there may be differences in the priorities people place on attaining this dream. For example, there are people who persevere despite the obstacles, disadvantages, and odds against them. There are others who do not persevere and who settle for some different version of the dream. This seems to suggest that despite the fact that there are similarities in aspirations between the working class and the middle and upper classes, we must look at the past history of these people. If someone has been a graduate student, then a course of treatment which includes long-term therapy geared toward the solution of the intrapsychic conflicts would seem reasonable because of the experience of long-term education. In contrast, a working-class person with less education may view such a proposal as being interminable, irrelevant, and financially impossible. This is an aspect that we need to consider. Although many people agree with the American Dream and speak of the importance of long-term therapy and the understanding of internal conflicts, we have to see if people place a high enough priority upon it to expand the necessary time and energy to accomplish it.

PROBLEMS IN TREATING POOR AND WORKING-CLASS PATIENTS

As we have suggested previously, therapists who have persevered and often sacrificed to obtain their education and occupation may have developed attitudes towards the poor and the working class which are covertly rejecting. Unwittingly, psychotherapists may fail to consider the needs of these patients, since most therapists have reached a higher plateau of life-style. This process of unconscious rejection or omission may be further compounded at times by several other factors.

For example, striving professional people may experience guilt feelings about primarily learning psychodynamic therapy with upper-middle-class patients when they see that the vast majority of patients belong to the working and the poor classes. To reject as unsuitable such a large proportion of patients may often pose a conflict for many well-intentioned therapists.

A second factor may be related to the American myth of the melting pot and the concept of equal status for all. According to the American ideology, virtually everyone should belong to the middle class and there should be no distinct differences between classes. However, this is not the reality and can pose dilemmas for those professionals who must deal with people of different classes. In order to compensate for conflicting feelings about social classes, the psychotherapist may react by being blind to the differences of the life-style of the working class and the poor, insisting fervently that all Americans belong to the middle class and that patients will respond to psychodynamic therapy only if they are suitable.

Psychotherapists who have immigrated to the United States may also have special problems. It is possible that some therapists may have been socialized with distinct social classes in other nations and so may have learned to behave with certain demeanors and attitudes toward individuals in social categories different than their own. These overt behaviors are usually not expected in the United States. Such behavior may include being peremptory, authoritarian, and directive with individuals in a lower class. Thus, the newly immigrated psychotherapist may unwittingly communicate to the patient a certain lack of respect for the patient's social status.

Because of the above situations, therapists from all backgrounds should guard against the following behaviors.

1. Using words that are too esoteric or abstract for the patient
2. Constantly interrupting the patient, without giving the patient enough of a chance to express himself or herself fully
3. Asking the patient questions with impatience and aggressiveness, rather than with true interest
4. Lecturing to the patient
5. Pretending to understand statements made by the patient when not truly understanding them, and not asking for clarification of what is said by the patient
6. Giving the patient a treatment plan, or an expectation for duration of treatment, without discussing it or negotiating it with the patient
7. Failing to use outside resources if such resources are necessary to help the patient cope with life problems
8. Not explaining the differences between psychotherapy and general medical treatment to the patient

Although these eight behaviors should be avoided in therapy with all patients, they are behaviors which are more easily and unintentionally committed when treating poor or working-class patients. Thus, a therapist must take special care to avoid the above pitfalls to effective therapy.

Now please complete the Self-Assessment Exercise 2.2.

SELF-ASSESSMENT EXERCISE 2.2

1. Describe the difference between the poor and working classes and the middle and upper classes regarding their use of mental health services.

2. Describe how sex and social class relate to the use of mental health services.

3. List eight behaviors which can damage the therapeutic relationship with a poor or working-class patient and therefore should be avoided.

When you have finished this exercise, check your answers with those that follow.

SELF-ASSESSMENT EXERCISE 2.2: FEEDBACK

1. In contrast to the middle and upper classes, the working class tend to need more encouragement to use mental health services appropriately and adequately. Without appropriate information and education, such patients tend to shy away from mental health services and seek the help of medical practitioners and other advisers instead.

2. Male and female professionals tend to use mental health services equally. Among the working class, the women tend to use the services slightly more frequently. This may be because it is more difficult for the male in the working class to get time off from work without losing income.

3. Behaviors to be avoided when providing psychotherapy for the poor and working class include

   a. Using words that are too esoteric or abstract for the patient
   b. Constantly interrupting the patient, without giving the patient enough of a chance to express himself or herself fully
   c. Asking the patient questions with impatience and aggressiveness, rather than with true interest
   d. Lecturing to the patient
   e. Pretending to understand statements made by the patient when not truly understanding them, and not asking for clarification of what is said by the patient
   f. Giving the patient a treatment plan, or an expectation for duration of treatment, without discussing it or negotiating it with the patient
   g. Failing to use outside resources if such resources are necessary to help the patient cope with life problems
   h. Not explaining the differences between psychotherapy and general medical treatment to the patient

If your answers correspond closely with those above, please continue reading. If not, please reread the preceding material.

EFFECTIVE THERAPEUTIC APPROACHES

Virtually all psychotherapeutic approaches may be included within four broad categories: psychotherapy, behavior therapy, pharmacological therapy, and environmental intervention. The therapies which seem to be of particular effectiveness will now be discussed within each of these categories.

Psychotherapy

The traditional long-term, verbal, nondirective psychotherapy is generally not appropriate, as it is typically taught, for the majority of poor or working-class patients. However, when modified to meet the specific needs of the patient, psychotherapy can be a valuable tool, particularly when the therapist shows an awareness of the environmental constraints and sociocultural factors, the needs and perspectives of the patient.

Setting time limits with your patient may facilitate therapy. Keep in mind that the average patient visits the clinic only four to six times. This figure is based on national averages for both private and public practice (Lorion, 1972). Much research is still needed to evaluate the effectiveness of time-limited therapy; but short-term goals often include symptom relief or problem solving.

Crisis intervention offers help that is brief, time-limited, and highly focused on quick and accurate identification of a crisis, its precipitating causes, and its high level of stress (Jacobson, 1974; Jacobson, Strickler, & Morley, 1968). It further helps the patient to identify and use available resources, personal strengths, and old and new coping behaviors. The crisis intervention approach was initially pioneered by Lindemann and Kaplan in the 1940s.

Role preparation for patients beginning therapy appears to show much promise. A number of studies with middle-class patients have shown encouraging results. Hoehn-Saric, Frank, Imber, Nash, Stone, & Battle (1964) used a role induction interview written by Orne and Wender (1968) to prepare patients for analytic therapy. Their results indicated that patients who were thus prepared showed more symptom reduction, and better attendance and social functioning than did patients who were not prepared. The implication was that developing more accurate expectations could lead to more effective use of analytic therapy. Several studies have replicated these positive results. More recently, Strupp and Bloxom (1973) developed a film showing the effectiveness of group therapy for a truck driver. Strupp and Bloxom found that patients who were presented with this film had better group attendance and more symptom reduction. Although long-term therapy as an initial approach may be appropriate for only a minority of poor and working-class patients, it may be indicated after the brief problem-solving approach has been implemented.

Behavior Therapy

Behavior therapy is characterized by the application of a variety of treatment paradigms which have their bases in learning and social-learning theories. Behavior therapy typically requires the therapist to actively engage in directing and teaching the patient how to change specific behaviors. The application of positive or negative reinforcers, rewards, or punishments, for example, is common in behavioral approaches to augment or to extinguish target behaviors. This approach often fits the patient's expectations of an active and directive therapist. For this reason it seems to have some specific value in the treatment of the poor and working-class patient (Goldstein, 1971).

One technique used in behavior therapy is assertiveness training. In this treatment method, patients are encouraged to stand up for their rights in a more appropriate fashion (Alberti & Emmons, 1974). This is clearly delineated from and contrasted to aggressive behavior, which may be threatening or negative in interpersonal relationships. Assertiveness training may be accomplished either individually or in groups. In our clinical experience, many of our low-income and working-class patients have benefited from some assertiveness training.

Another example of the behavioral approach is the use of desensitization with phobic patients. In the classical technique of Wolpe (1958), a hierarchy of fear stimuli is established, ranging from the most threatening to the least threatening image for the patient. These stimuli are successively presented to the patient while the patient is in a state of deep relaxation. The relaxation is learned through muscular exercises which are modifications of Jacobson's technique of progressive relaxation. Desensitization techniques require a great deal of therapist guidance and interaction with the patient.

Modeling is another frequently used behavioral approach. The therapist may serve as a positive example in modeling a behavior which is to be encouraged, for example, speaking to a feared person. The patient may then be encouraged to follow the example and to behave in ways that cope with specific problems.

Behavioral approaches may be especially useful with working-class and poor patients because in contrast to traditional long-term treatment, behavioral approaches are often designed for specific and limited time intervals. For example, brief treatment over 10 to 12 sessions has been used for the diminution of phobic symptoms and sexual dysfunction. The patient can thus see symptomatic relief quickly and often has a clearer understanding of what is expected in therapy.

Pharmacological Therapy

Medications should be prescribed for such disorders as anxiety, depression, and psychosis as indicated, regardless of class. Caution needs to be exercised with patients who do not have adequate social support systems immediately available to them. Where they are inadequate, the therapist may seek institutional support on a temporary basis. For example, chronic patients who need long-term treatments (schizophrenia and manic-depressive disorders) can be placed in a board-and-care facility and needed treatment can be given by the staff. Many patients may drop out of treatment unless they are convinced of its necessity and unless relatives and others are cooperative. Keep in mind that all of us tend to discontinue medication if we feel well, have side effects, or are distracted by other demands.

Environmental Intervention

Patients will require assistance with problems of living as well as with emotional problems. It is therefore often necessary to engage the assistance of community workers, community aides, and medical case workers. These paraprofessionals have areas of expertise and are willing to help in this aspect of therapy. Their effectiveness is often linked to the degree of training that they have received, to their personality and interests, and to their understanding of and upbringing in the community which they are serving. Their identification with the people they serve is critical.

Paraprofessionals can be of service in a number of ways. For example, if someone needs placement in a board-and-care home, the medical case worker can often help with the referral. Similarly, if the patient is having problems dealing with some real issue involving social service or other agencies in the community, the community workers might be willing to go out with the patient and try to help him arrive at some appropriate resolution of his problems. If there are medical problems, as are more frequent among working-class and poor patients, it would be appropriate to refer the patient for concomitant medical care.

Many other possible avenues exist for individualized environmental intervention. The key for therapists to remember is that, despite the stereotypes, each patient needs individualized treatment planning.

Now please complete the Self-Assessment Exercise 2.3.

SELF-ASSESSMENT EXERCISE 2.3

Outline the approach which seems to be most effective with the poor and the working-class patient within each of the following therapy categories:

1. Psychotherapy

2. Behavior therapy

3. Pharmacological therapy

4. Environmental intervention

When you have completed this exercise, check your answers with those that follow.

SELF-ASSESSMENT EXERCISE 2.3: FEEDBACK

The approaches that seem to be most effective with poor and working-class patients are as follows:

1. Psychotherapy
   Time-limited and problem-oriented psychotherapy which is delivered with an understanding of the patient's entire environment, sociocultural background, and current status, has proven to be effective with poor and working-class patients.

2. Behavior therapy
   Such treatment paradigms as the application of reward or punishment of specific behaviors seem to fit the patient's expectations of an active and authoritative therapist. Examples of specific behavioral approaches include assertiveness training, desensitization, and modeling.

3. Pharmacological therapy
   Medications should be prescribed for the poor and working-class patient as for the middle- or upper-class patient. Care must be taken to insure that a cooperative support group is available.

4. Environmental intervention
   Direct intervention into the social and working activities of these patients is necessary to correct their emotional and living problems.

If your answers correspond closely with those above, please continue reading. If not, please reread the preceding materials.

SUMMARY

Nearly 70% of all citizens of the United States belong to the poor or working class (Hollingshead & Redlich, 1958). The most effective therapy for these patients may be conceptualized in brief segments of time from four to six sessions at most. With this brief treatment preconception in mind, the therapist will be much more aware of the possible times when the patient might be actively helped.

The key to effective therapy is flexibility. The therapist must respond as if each session may possibly be the last one (Yamamoto & Goin, 1965). Our patients expect therapy to be brief, to involve active counseling by the therapist which is directed toward the relief of specific problems or symptoms (Baum & Felzer, 1964). Some patients will need longer-term therapy (individual, group, family) after a period of individual preparation. Flexibility and an individualized approach with due consideration for the patient's needs and expectations will often be successful.

REFERENCES

Alberti, R. E., & Emmons, M. L. *Your perfect right* (2nd. ed.). San Luis Obispo, Calif.: Impact Publishers, 1974.

Allen, V. L. *Psychological factors in poverty.* Chicago: Markham, 1970.

Baum, O. E., & Felzer, S. Activity in initial interviews with lower-class patients. *Archives of General Psychiatry,* 1964, *10,* 345–353.

Coleman, R. P., & Rainwater, L. *Social standing in America.* New York: Basic Books, 1978.

Dohrenwend, B. P., & Dohrenwend, B. S. Social and cultural influences on psychopathology. *Annual Review of Psychology,* 1974, *25,* 417–452.

Fishman, J. R. Poverty, race and violence. *American Journal of Psychotherapy,* 1969, *23,* 599–607.

Frank, A., Eisenthal, S., & Lazare, A. Are there social class differences in patient treatment conceptions? *Archives of General Psychiatry,* 1978, *35,* 61–69.

Goldstein, A. P. *Psychotherapeutic attraction.* New York: Pergamon, 1971.

Gould, R. E. Dr. Strangeclass: Or how I stopped worrying about the theory and began treating the blue-collar worker. *American Journal of Orthopsychiatry,* 1967, *37,* 78–86.

Hill, R. B. *The strength of black families.* New York: Emerson Hall, 1971.

Hoehn-Saric, R., Frank, J. D., Imber, S. D., Nash, E. H., Stone, A. R., & Battle, C. C. Systematic preparation of patients for psychotherapy: I. Effects on therapy behavior and outcome. *Journal of Psychiatric Research,* 1964, *2,* 267–281.

Hollingshead, A. B., & Redlich, F. C. *Social class and mental illness: A community study.* New York: Wiley, 1958.

Jacobson, G. F. Programs and techniques of crisis intervention. In G. Caplan (Ed.), *American handbook of psychiatry* (Vol. 2). New York: Basic Books, 1974.

Jacobson, G. F., Strickler, M., & Morley, W. Generic and individual approaches to crisis intervention. *American Journal of Public Health,* 1968, *58,* 338–343.

Lorion, R. P. *Social class differences in treatment attitudes and expectations.* Unpublished doctoral dissertation, University of Rochester, 1972.

Orne, M. T., & Wender, P. H. Anticipatory socialization for psychotherapy: Method and rationale. *American Journal of Psychiatry,* 1968, *124,* 88–98.

President's Commission on Mental Health. *Report to the President* (Vol. 1). Washington, D.C.: U.S. Government Printing Office, 1978.

Redlich, F., & Kellert, S. Trends in American mental health. *American Journal of Psychiatry,* 1978, *135,* 22–28.

Srole, L., Langer, T. S., Michael, S. T., Opler, M. K., & Rennie, T. A. C. *Mental health in the metropolis: The Midtown Manhattan study.* New York: McGraw-Hill, 1962.

Strupp, H., & Bloxom, A. L. Preparing lower-class patients for group psychotherapy:

Development and evaluation of a role-induction film. *Journal of Consulting and Clinical Psychology*, 1973, *41*, 373–384.

Thomas, A., & Sillen, S. *Racism and psychiatry*. New York: Brunner/Mazel, 1972.

U.S. Bureau of Census. *Statistical abstracts of the United States: 1974* (95th ed.). Washington, D.C.: U.S. Government Printing Office, 1974.

Wolpe, J. *Psychotherapy by reciprocal inhibition*. Stanford: Stanford University Press, 1958.

Yamamoto, J., & Goin, M. On the treatment of the poor. *American Journal of Psychiatry*, 1965, *122*, 267–271.

CHAPTER 3

The Hispanic-American Patient

Frank X. Acosta and Leonard A. Evans

INTRODUCTION

This chapter will discuss sociocultural characteristics of the Hispanic community and show how these characteristics relate to mental health and mental health services. Specific recommendations for treatment approaches and psychotherapy will also be presented. It is important to focus on Hispanic Americans because they constitute the second largest minority group in the United States and the fastest growing ethnic group in our country (Russell & Satterwhite, 1978). It is of further importance since Hispanic Americans in our country have been severely underserved by mental health facilities (Acosta, 1977; Padilla, Ruiz, & Alvarez, 1975; President's Commission on Mental Health, 1978).

The special purpose of this chapter is to present an overview of the unique problems and limitations experienced by psychotherapists in treating Hispanic Americans and describe some of the ways of resolving these problems.

After completing this chapter and a corresponding group discussion session, the reader should be able to:

1. Describe the sociocultural characteristics of Hispanic Americans which may affect the service they receive at a mental health facility
2. Describe the important attitudes of Hispanic Americans toward mental health services
3. Discuss the most common problems faced by therapists when treating Hispanic Americans

4. Describe and use therapeutic approaches which are most effective with Hispanic Americans
5. Experience satisfaction with the process and outcome of therapeutic encounters with Hispanic Americans

Please read the above learning objectives until you become familiar with the goals of this chapter; then begin reading the following section.

CHARACTERISTICS OF HISPANIC AMERICANS

Demographics

Spanish-surnamed Americans have been typically under-counted because of inaccurate census procedures, such as failure to provide enough bilingual interviewers (Hernandez, Estrada, & Alvirez, 1973). Currently available census figures show the Hispanic population to number 12 million (U.S. Bureau of the Census, 1980). The following are the available census breakdowns of Hispanic groups: Mexican American, 7.2 million; Puerto Rican, 1.8 million; and Spanish, 3.0 million, which includes persons of Central or South American, Cuban, and other Spanish origin (U.S. Bureau of the Census, 1980). Although these 1980 figures do not provide a further breakdown for the category "Spanish," an indication of the potential breakdown for "Spanish" may be derived from the 1974 census figures which then showed a total Hispanic population of 9.1 million with: Mexican American, 5.0 million; Puerto Rican, 1.5 million; Central and South American, 0.5 million; Cuban, 0.6 million, and other Spanish origin, 1.5 million (U.S. Bureau of the Census, 1974).

The estimates reported here are probably very conservative. In discussing the difficulty of estimating the Hispanic population, Le-Vine and Padilla (1980) have noted, for example, that beyond the figures provided by the 1975 U.S. Bureau of the Census report, other estimates were providing numbers which ranged from 4.8 million to 12.2 million higher than the 11.2 million estimates reported in 1975. These much higher figures were including census undercount, legal immigration, and undocumented immigrants.

In Los Angeles County alone, the population of the Hispanic community is 2.0 million or 28.7% of Los Angeles County's entire population (Los Angeles County, 1978). This figure represents a significant Hispanic growth in Los Angeles County from 18.3% in 1970 to 28.7% in 1978. Indeed, 45% of all births in Los Angeles County in 1977 were to Spanish surname parents (Los Angeles County, 1978).

The majority of Hispanic Americans are in the low-income and poor socioeconomic level (U.S. Bureau of Census, 1974). They are also severely underrepresented in higher levels of education, occupation, and professional ranking (Grebler, Moore, & Guzman, 1970; U.S. Bureau of the Census, 1980).

Culture

Heritage. Hispanic Americans are also known as Chicanos, *latinos,* Mexicanos, *hispanos,* Spanish-speaking Americans, Spanish Americans, and Spanish-surnamed Americans. A considerable number of these names were coined by government officials and popularized.

The heritage of Hispanic Americans is rich and diverse. Some commonalities do exist, however, such as shared lineage with both Spanish and local indigenous Indian groups.

A brief description of the heritage of Mexican Americans offers some insights into Hispanic culture. Historically, Mexican Americans are descendants of Indians, Mexicans and Spaniards who lived in the area now known as the Southwestern United States before the American colonies were formed. A fair number of Mexican Americans residing in New Mexico, for example, identify themselves as *hispanos* or Spanish Americans, and thus place significant emphasis on their Spanish roots. On the other hand, a growing number of both young and old Mexican Americans throughout the United States now identify themselves as Chicanos. The name Chicano suggests a proud sense of Mexican, Indian, and Spanish heritage and of social and political unity. At present the most commonly used self-identification still appears to be Mexican American (Acosta & Sheehan, 1976; Padilla, Carlos, & Keefe, 1976).

The present-day Mexican-American culture is a unique product of cultural fusions that began its most dramatic white-Indian blending process in the 16th century. It was in the early 1500s that Hernando Cortes led his group of Spanish explorers to overtake and almost decimate the well-established Aztec empire in central Mexico. A great deal of intermarriage between Spaniards and Indians resulted over the next several hundred years, as did the mixing of Spanish traditions, language, and Catholicism with Indian customs, teachings, and beliefs.

Since several thousand years B.C. Mexico had experienced such advanced Indian civilizations as the Olmecs, the Teotihuacános, the Toltecs, the Mayas, the Mixtecs, and the Aztecs. The impact of these civilizations is still evident throughout Mexico. In fact, outside of the urban areas a large number of Indian groups and tribes still maintain their life-styles and languages.

The Mexican-American culture today is still an evolving process, one which incorporates the heritage of past Indian and Spanish cultures and the more recent Anglo-American and modern Mexican cultures.

Much heterogeneity exists among Mexican Americans and other Hispanic Americans in terms of their sociocultural characteristics. Therefore, it is important for therapists to know their patients' ethnic self-identity, language, religion, family ties, and acculturation.

Language. Spanish is the native language used in the homes of more than half the Hispanic population (U.S. Bureau of Census, 1974). An even greater number probably understand or speak some Spanish. It is common, for example, for second- or third-generation Hispanic Americans to understand Spanish well, but they may speak only a little.

A wide variation thus exists in the degree of English- or Spanish-language fluency and in the degree of bilingualism among Hispanic Americans. It is common in the *barrios*, or communities, for people to speak to each other in both English and Spanish.

The attitude of the general American public has usually been negative toward people who cannot speak English. Such people are often considered "dumb," "lazy," or "inferior." Psychotherapists sometimes harbor similar attitudes.

Many problems arise in therapy with patients who speak only Spanish or broken English when therapists are not Spanish-speaking or bilingual. Several studies now show that bilingual patients have difficulty in expressing nuances of feeling and of fully disclosing problems and emotional states if they are not able to speak in their dominant language (Marcos & Alpert, 1976).

Family. Even today in the era of zero population growth, Hispanic Americans show higher rates of childbirth and younger mean ages

($\bar{X}$ = 18 years) than the general population ($\bar{X}$ = 28 years) (U.S. Bureau of Census, 1974). This results from the fact that the family has traditionally been one of the most valued and proud aspects of life among Hispanic Americans. A great deal of importance has typically been placed on preserving family unity, respect, and loyalty, and the family tends to be a source of strength for Hispanic Americans (Murillo, 1971; Padilla, Carlos, & Keefe, 1976; Penalosa, 1968).

The family structure is usually hierarchical with special respect and much authority given to the husband and father. The wife and mother is often obedient to her husband and also receives respect and much emotional reward from the children (Penalosa, 1968). Sex-role identification for the Hispanic American is thus much stricter than that of the general population of the United States. However, many of these traditional sex-role characteristics may also be found among the poor and the rural in our country. As Hispanic Americans move up the socioeconomic ladder to more middle-class levels and as more assimilation of Anglo life-styles occurs, sex-role delineations become less strict.

Interesting child-rearing patterns which reflect Hispanic-American parental attitudes have been described using the dimensions of cooperation versus competition and achievement aspirations. Kagan and Buriel (1977), for example, have demonstrated in a number of studies that Mexican and Mexican-American children show greater cooperation in a variety of tasks, while Anglo-American children show greater competitiveness. Again, the typical Hispanic-American family tends to stress unity and helpfulness to its members. While cooperation seems to be an important characteristic, achievement for their children is also encouraged by Hispanic-American parents (Grebler et al., 1970).

Hispanic Americans further tend to maintain extended family ties. These family connections and the frequency of contact among members tend to be greater than those of Anglo-Americans (Padilla et al., 1976). The extended family often includes both the immediate family and relatives, lifelong friends, and kin created through a Catholic baptismal custom, whereby the child acquires a godmother (*madrina*) and godfather (*padrino*), who directly share responsibility for the child's welfare and thus form coparent bonds with the child's parents as comother (*comadre*) and cofather (*compadre*).

It is important for therapists to be aware of family strengths and weaknesses, expectations and traditions, when providing therapeutic interventions. Family members should be included whenever possible to help select and implement treatment interventions. Many of the problems experienced by Hispanic patients are family related. For example, a patient may be despondent about being geographically separated from his or her family; or Hispanic women may experience marital conflicts if they do not accept traditional sex-role proscriptions; or parents and adolescents may experience not only the stresses of generation gap but also of cultural differences fostered by the adolescents' fuller assimilation experiences.

Cultural Ties. A large proportion of the Hispanic Americans in this country have parents who were born in Spanish-speaking countries or were themselves born in these countries. These close ties to another country often create a delay in the Hispanic American's assimilation in the United States.

Religion. Catholicism is the predominant religion for Hispanic Americans. This can be a strong resource in times of stress and illness. Prayer is often used even among Catholics who do not practice their religion. For about 95% of Mexican Americans, the religion of preference is Catholic (Grebler *et al.*, 1970).

Children are typically brought up to have strong beliefs in the existence of God, the importance of prayer, and regular participation in the mass or worship service. The neighborhood church and its priests and nuns are held in high esteem and serve as a valuable mechanism for community worship and moral support.

With adolescence and adulthood, many male Hispanic Americans tend to lose the regularity of their religious practice but do maintain some church attendance and their religious beliefs. Women tend to be the most visible and active members of the church. It is reasonable to assume that in times of stress, fear, and confusion, many Mexican Americans turn to both private and community prayer for support.

Catholic philosophy and religious practices may affect Hispanic-American patient expectations and participation in psychotherapy. For example, Catholic precepts argue that it is helpful for one's eternal salvation to sacrifice in this world, to be charitable to others, to be able to endure wrongs done against you, to remain free from sin, to be Christ-like, and to place more importance on one's spiritual dimensions than on the acquisition of material goods. This pattern will often make it more difficult for a patient to speak up or to be more assertive during a therapy session. Catholic patients may also be more accustomed to seeing a priest for the sacrament of confession. Through this practice an individual privately confesses all sins or wrongdoings to a priest and usually receives immediate absolution or forgiveness after an expression of genuine penitence. Some Catholic patients may thus see a therapist in a priest's role and anticipate some kind of immediate help.

Thus it is important for therapists to gain an understanding of their patients' religious beliefs and practices, and how these beliefs and experiences may facilitate or counteract therapy. It may also be important for therapists to consult with or to refer their patient to a priest or minister on those occasions when a priest's intervention would seem particularly necessary as in the following cases.

CASE HISTORY

José

José, a young 35-year-old Spanish-speaking Mexican, came to the clinic complaining of trembling in his hands, sweating, and shortness of breath. He appeared to be a strong and straightforward individual. He stated that his work performance as an upholsterer had been deteriorating for several months. His major conflict focused on his wish to marry his girlfriend and the resulting need to decrease the amount of money he was sending to his parents and younger brothers and sisters in Mexico. He felt he would be committing a crime or a sin if he were to reduce his help to his family. He had sought advice in the mental health clinic because he thought he was going crazy. He had never experienced such sudden onsets of anxiety before. In addition to helping this patient express his feelings and his needs in short-term therapy, the therapist encouraged him to speak to a priest about his fears of committing a sin against his family. José did consult with a priest over several meetings and also completed eight sessions of short-term therapy. His anxiety diminished, his work improved, and he decided to propose marriage to his girlfriend when therapy ended.

When Hispanic patients, such as José, seek help with problems which center on their self-criticism and guilt for not having done enough for others, we assess their level of religious involvement and determine if therapy alone will be sufficient or if the patient should also consult with a priest. In many cases, the priest's consultation is critical to lowering patients' felt level of guilt for their shortcomings.

It would also be important for therapists in treating sexual dysfunctions, or patients' concerns with sexual feelings or behaviors in general, to assess the effects of any therapeutic interventions on patients' own religious beliefs. Hispanic patients may unexpectedly terminate therapy if the therapist shows a disregard for their own beliefs and attitudes in the treatment plans which the therapist prescribes.

In cases of bereavement, we have seen Hispanic patients suffering through their grief and showing signs of reactive depression who tell us that their main strength is prayer. In other cases, we have seen Hispanic patients who are suffering through bereavement and who have lost contact with their priest or minister.

Lupe

Lupe was a 38-year-old Spanish-speaking Mexican-American woman. Her husband was stabbed to death while defending a friend in a *barrio* poolroom. Two months after the tragedy, Lupe was referred to our mental health clinic by her family because they felt she was becoming more depressed and *estraña* (strange). Her symptoms included a 10-pound weight loss, insomnia, crying, and chest pains in the area in which her husband had been stabbed. Her depression was fairly normal for the gravity of her loss, and she was reassured by knowing that she wasn't going *loca* (crazy). She was able to maintain her household and care for her four children.

Lupe contracted for six sessions of crisis intervention and six sessions of group therapy. In addition, she was advised to consult with her parish priest and became involved in a church volunteer program. She stated that both her therapy and her involvement in her church had helped her a great deal. She was able to sleep better, and her chest pains greatly diminished. At the end of her therapy plan, Lupe requested to continue in group therapy for an additional six sessions to gain further support from the group members.

Social Interactions

Discrimination. Unlike many other ethnic groups who undergo the process of assimilation into the general United States culture and in the process often experience a short duration of discrimination (Stonequist, 1961), Hispanic Americans have been longtime victims of discrimination in our country (Grebler *et al.*, 1970). One of the effects of discrimination against a group is that it can lower the group's own sense of self-esteem, self-identity, and hope. In a study by Dworkin (1965), for example, it was found that a group of native-born low-income Mexican Americans held significantly more negative attitudes about themselves than a comparison group of foreign-born low-income Mexican Americans. These findings suggest that the longer years of discrimination suffered by the native-born resulted in lowered levels of self-pride and self-esteem.

Discrimination has in general been subtle and rejecting; overt discrimination against Hispanic Americans was never sanctioned by this country's laws as it was for blacks. Nonetheless, countless numbers of Hispanic Americans have felt the sting of being second- or third-class citizens. Hispanic Americans, for example, often feel excluded from active and important roles in government, television, radio, or newspapers, even though they feel fully qualified to fill these roles.

Recently, the dramatic Los Angeles play *Zoot Suit*, by Luis Valdez, poignantly re-enacted the false murder conviction of 17 Chicano youths and the zoot-suit riots which occurred in Los Angeles in 1943. A main point stressed in this play was the open and accepted discrimination shown by the press and the legal system against the Chicano youths.

It may be that Hispanic Americans' strong preservation of the Spanish language, their dominant brown skin tones, and their Spanish surnames have earmarked them more than other ethnic groups for continued discrimination.

Acculturation. Within the Hispanic-American community there is a wide range in the degree of acculturation. Some Hispanic Americans have a very close identity with the culture of their families; others identify with the Anglo-American culture. The acculturation process leads to increased states of psychological stress as explained in the following illustrations:

1. For recent immigrants, integrating one's ethnic identity into a new culture is difficult and may lead to denial, depression, or avoidance of one's ethnic identity.
2. Adopting new value systems that may clash with or contradict old ones is stressful.
3. Developing a positive self-identity is more difficult for a youth

who must identify with two distinct cultural groups simultaneously.

4. For many immigrants, becoming part of the poor class in a new country is almost inevitable if the person has few skills, little education, and little or no money.

5. Individuals in the process of acculturation are more subject to stereotypes and discrimination because of their different-ness from the majority culture.

6. An incomplete or marginal state of acculturation, neither re-jecting nor accepting a new culture and value system, causes its own level of stress. For example, Fabrega and Wallace (1968) found that this state correlated with more serious types of disorders among hospitalized groups of Mexican Ameri-cans. The pressures of discrimination and acculturation affect the mental health of the Mexican American person. A number of studies have already indicated that low-income and de-prived people are more subject to higher states of psycholog-ical stress (Hollingshead & Redlich, 1958; Srole, Langer, Mi-chael, Opler, & Rennie, 1962). The combinations of socioeconomic deficits and acculturation pressures almost as-sure a high need for mental health services among Hispanic Americans (Acosta, 1979).

Now complete the Self-Assessment Exercise 3.1.

SELF-ASSESSMENT EXERCISE 3.1

1. Discuss the following cultural characteristics and how they may affect the service the Hispanic-American patient receives in a mental health outpatient center.

   a. Spanish language

   b. Family structure

   c. Cultural ties

   d. Catholic religion

2. Discuss the following social interactions and how they may affect the service the Hispanic-American patient receives in a mental health outpatient center.

   a. Discrimination

   b. Acculturation

When you have completed this exercise, check your answers with those that follow.

SELF-ASSESSMENT EXERCISE 3.1: FEEDBACK

1. The following cultural characteristics may affect the service the Hispanic-American patient receives in a mental health outpatient center.

   a. Spanish language
   Spanish is the native language of the majority of Hispanic-American patients; English fluency varies considerably. Unless the therapist is Spanish-speaking or bilingual, communication can suffer.

   b. Family structure
   Family and extended family members are very close. It may be possible to enlist family members to support the patient's treatment.

   c. Cultural ties
   A significant number of Hispanic Americans have very close cultural ties with Spanish-speaking countries. Knowing the patients' cultural traditions will assist the therapist in treating these patients.

   d. Catholic religion
   The Catholic religion is the most popular religion for the Hispanic American. The importance of prayer and the value placed upon stoicism by these patients will influence the therapist's understanding of the behavior of these patients.

2. Discuss the following social interactions and how they may affect the service the Hispanic-American patient receives in a mental health outpatient center.

   a. Discrimination
   Long-standing discrimination can cause low self-esteem; this is frequently found in the Hispanic-American patient. This aspect of the patient's personality may require a great deal of attention during therapy. There may also be fear of experiencing discrimination by white mental health professionals.

   b. Acculturation
   The process of dealing with one's original culture while attempting to live in a new culture causes much anxiety. People in this position often have little money, find it hard to get jobs, are discriminated against, and therefore may require psychological and environmental support. Self-identity is often affected by the process of acculturation among ethnic minority group members. This problem should be considered and ruled out or dealt with.

If your answers correspond closely with those above, please continue reading. If not, please reread the preceding material.

ATTITUDES TOWARD MENTAL HEALTH SERVICES

In general, Hispanic Americans, like many Americans in the United States, are more accustomed to seeing general physicians rather than mental health professionals for emotional problems (Padilla *et al.*, 1976). Thus, many patients who do arrive at a mental health facility may be unclear about the kind of treatment that they can receive. These patients may well be expecting more traditional medical help. For example, some of our patients have openly asked why we were not taking blood tests in the first interview. In spite of this lack of awareness, several community survey and research studies have shown that Hispanic Americans have a high positive regard for counseling and psychotherapy (Acosta & Sheehan, 1976; Karno & Edgarton, 1969).

Once in therapy, Hispanic-American patients will probably not disagree readily with therapists about anything, even when such disagreement may be warranted. This is because therapists are perceived as authority figures.

Studies indicate that the Spanish-speaking, Spanish-surnamed patients who do seek mental health services typically receive less and briefer forms of therapy than do Anglo-American patients (Karno, 1966; Padilla *et al.*, 1975; Sue, 1977; Yamamoto, James, Bloombaum, & Hattem, 1967). It is not yet established if the therapy received is briefer because of therapist or patient decisions.

Rates of initial therapy utilization are also low (Acosta, 1977; 1979). It is noteworthy, however, that clinics which have large bilingual, bicultural Spanish staff show higher rates of utilization by Hispanic Americans (Heiman, Burruel, & Chavez, 1975; Karno & Morales, 1971).

There appear to be several main reasons why Hispanic Americans have low mental health service utilization rates even though they have a generally high regard for such services. These reasons include:

1. Language differences between non–Spanish-speaking therapists and Spanish-speaking patients
2. Social class and cultural differences between therapists and patients
3. Insufficient number of mental health facilities (bilingual or not) in the *barrios*

4. Wide use of physicians for primary help with psychological problems
5. Tendency of Hispanic-American patients to wait a long time before seeking mental health help
6. Lack of awareness of the existence of mental health clinics

Folk healers (*curanderos, espiritistas*) are sometimes, but not often, called on for help with mental health problems. They rely primarily on herbs, massage, diets, advice, prayer, suggestion, and persuasion in helping individuals with physical or psychological problems. Experienced and trained folk healers may have a wide repertoire of treatments for different ailments. In cases where individuals present with psychosomatic problems and hold a high belief in the treatment and curative abilities of the folk healer, successful interventions may be possible. Such presenting problems as stomach disorders and recurring headaches may be treated by special diets and reassurance.

The use of folk healers is probably more common in rural and small communities in Spanish-speaking countries but appears to be sporadic and sketchy in the United States. There appears to be wider use of folk healers in parts of Texas (Kiev, 1968), for example, than in California (Edgarton, Karno, & Fernandez, 1970).

Our own experience with Hispanic-American patients indicates that only a few patients out of many have sought the help of folk healers for psychological problems and have done so even while involved in psychotherapy. These patients have typically returned to therapy and report little to no symptom changes as a result of the *curandero's* intervention. Nonetheless, patients who do not return to therapy may have been helped, since some patients have reported hearing of folk healers who are highly regarded and who are visited by individuals in psychological stress.

PROBLEMS IN TREATING HISPANIC-AMERICAN PATIENTS

Developing Patient Trust

Some Hispanic Americans may find difficulty in trusting a therapist. Because Hispanic Americans have often experienced discrimination and quiet nonresponsiveness from the majority system, they may view the therapist as a representative of the system. Because of their past experiences, patients may initially find it hard to believe that the therapist is interested in them. This is doubly true of Hispanics who are in the United States without documents because they may fear being reported to the immigration service by the therapist. In such a case, the therapist should explain that he has no intentions of reporting the patient and that all matters discussed will be kept strictly confidential. Thus, it is important that therapists show interest and a willingness to help, if such help is appropriate, and encourage their patients to confide.

Treating the Non–English-Speaking Patient

There is an obvious problem when a non–Spanish-speaking therapist attempts to treat a Spanish-speaking patient. An immediate impasse will be reached. Often therapists will call on the help of untrained bilingual staff or relatives to help them interpret. However, the use of untrained and unsupervised interpreters may lead to a number of translating problems, such as language distortions, editing, and deletions. In these difficult situations it would be advisable for non–Spanish-speaking therapists to employ the help of trained interpreters or to consult with a Spanish-speaking therapist.

It would be highly useful to speak some Spanish with patients who favor speaking in Spanish, even though they may be bilingual. A caution, however: The therapist should not use Spanish in an impatient or forced fashion but only out of sincere interest in and expression of friendliness to the patient.

Many popularly used words and phrases could be taught to therapists within the clinical setting. It would also be most helpful for mental health facilities to provide comprehensive glossaries and dictionaries in Spanish and English of both basic language and psychological concepts (e.g., Velasquez, Gray, & Iribas, 1974). Therapists would thus be equipped with some basic language tools to assist in the therapy of Spanish-speaking patients.

In lieu of bilingual staff, trained bilingual interpreters may be of valuable assistance to therapists. The result of a study by Kline, Acosta, Austin, and Johnson (1980) indicated that Spanish-speaking patients who were interviewed through the help of an interpreter felt greatly understood and were positive about their treatment experience; interestingly, they were even more positive than were bilingual patients who did not need the help of an interpreter and spoke to a therapist directly in English. In striking contrast to these findings, the non–Spanish-speaking therapists felt that the patients who had been evaluated through the help of an interpreter did not want to return, did not feel understood, and did not feel that they had received any help. The two perceptions were thus incongruent. The implications of this study are that the therapists may have projected onto the patients their own possible sense of discomfort, insecurity and general uncertainty in their data base. This is created by a loss of their own sense of precision in relying on someone else. On the other hand, the Spanish-speaking patients may have expressed even greater positivity than their bilingual counterparts as part of their appreciation for receiving better than usual attention from non–Spanish-speaking therapists who were assisted by skilled interpreters.

The impact and success of trained bilingual interpreters in a community clinic has been reported (Acosta, 1977, 1979; Acosta & Cristo, 1981). Greater and more comprehensive services can be offered to Spanish-speaking patients with the help of trained bilingual interpreters when the majority of therapists are non–Spanish-speaking.

Cultural Differences between Therapist and Patient

Therapists often come from or achieve middle- or upper-middle-class status. They are rarely of Hispanic-American background. These patient–therapist differences and the consequent lack of knowledge of each other's culture and social status can lead to lack of understanding, strife, and dissatisfaction with the therapy process on the part of both patient and therapist.

For example, if the patient is a woman from a traditional Mexican family, and if the family ties are still close to Mexico, it may be important for the therapist to ask the patient if the dominant male member of the family could be consulted with about the overall treatment plan. Further, it would be important to explore the patient's feelings about this consultation. It should be recognized that the male could prevent any continued treatment if he feels he doesn't know what is going on and doesn't have a role. It may be important and even necessary, to include him and the entire family in the consultation and in the therapy.

It is important to use community resources and workers whenever possible. Such resources, for example, include vocational rehabilitation and training, employment counseling, legal aid, and financial assistance. As is true in the mental health system, community services are often lacking for the Spanish-speaking patient. It may take additional effort for therapists to mobilize community services to assist the Spanish-speaking patient.

It is important to show a sense of personal interest, that is, friendliness and warmth, in the Hispanic-American patient (Casavantes, 1975). This interest can be shown by determining the cultural background and the social and developmental history of the patient. Is the patient first, second, third, or fourth generation? Recently arrived from Mexico, or from a Central or South American country, or from Puerto Rico, or Cuba? From a small community or a large city? Is the patient managing the acculturation process well? What role does religion have in the patient's life?

It is of particular importance to explain the value of therapy to male Hispanic-American patients, because their cultures stress the concept that men must be strong and stoic. It must be explained that it is not a sign of weakness or inferiority to openly discuss personal problems with a therapist.

It is important to be sensitive to the kind of language that you use. Language should not be too sophisticated. This is particularly true if the patient's English vocabulary is not as advanced as the therapist's.

In addition to helping patients with intrapsychic difficulties, it is important to guide patients to deal with problems in their life, their community, and their environment, especially if it is suppressive. It is important to be aware of the patients' environmental constraints, which may be a determining factor in the continuation of therapy.

A number of Hispanic patients arrive at mental health facilities with high degrees of somatization. This may be due to the stresses they are facing, waiting too long to seek psychotherapy, or primarily visiting general physicians for essentially emotional problems. Although clear experimental data do not yet exist, clinical experience indicates that Hispanic Americans show a higher degree of somatization than do other patient groups. If this is the case with a particular patient, it is important to explain the problem of somatizing and emphasize the need to discuss personal problems openly in order to eliminate the somatic problems. The patient may need medication temporarily to provide more immediate elimination of some symptoms.

Now complete the Self-Assessment Exercise 3.2.

SELF-ASSESSMENT EXERCISE 3.2

1. Describe the general attitude of the Hispanic American toward mental health services.

2. List six reasons why the Hispanic-American people have low mental health services utilization rates.

3. Discuss the problem a therapist has in developing a Hispanic-American patient's trust. Then discuss possible solutions.

4. Discuss the problem an English-speaking therapist has when treating a Spanish-speaking patient. Then discuss possible solutions.

5. Discuss the problem of cultural differences between a therapist and a Hispanic-American patient in the following.

   a. Sex-role identification

b. Community resources

c. Personal interest

d. Somatization

When you have completed this exercise to the best of your ability, please check your answers with those that follow.

SELF-ASSESSMENT EXERCISE 3.2: FEEDBACK

1. Hispanic Americans generally regard mental health therapists highly; however, they have little knowledge of the process of psychotherapy and when to seek it.

2. Hispanic Americans have low mental health services utilization rates because of: language differences; social class and cultural differences; insufficient number of clinics in the *barrios*; wide use of physicians for emotional problems; waiting too long to seek help; and lack of awareness of available services.

3. A past history of discrimination and failure often makes patients distrustful of authority figures such as therapists. Sincere interest and encouragement on the part of the therapist is necessary to develop the trust of the patient.

4. The problem of communicating with a person who does not speak the same language is obvious. This problem is compounded when the source of the communication is feelings and beliefs. The situation may be helped by using bilingual therapists or trained interpreters, or by having therapists learn a selected list of Spanish words which commonly occur during psychotherapy.

5. Problems arising out of sociocultural differences may include:

   a. Sex-role identification
      The dominant male in the family may have to be consulted or included in therapy of family members.

   b. Community resources
      These resources are often missing or are difficult to mobilize for Hispanic-American patients. Special effort is often required.

   c. Personal interest
      Because of the history of discrimination and rejection, therapists must make a special effort to let Hispanic-American patients know that they are sincerely interested in their well-being.

   d. Somatization
      The special stresses placed on the Hispanic-American patient often cause psychosomatic complaints. Special inquiry is necessary to uncover these "hidden" causes of somatic complaints. Much explanation is necessary to help the patient understand the somatization process.

If your answers correspond closely with those above, please continue reading. If not, please reread the preceding material.

EFFECTIVE THERAPEUTIC APPROACHES

Psychotherapy

Educating Patients. It is important to explain your treatment plan to the patient, that is, what you are planning to do, what is expected of the patient, and approximately how long this plan will take to implement. Be as specific as possible regarding how many weeks, months, or years. The patient should be encouraged to let the therapist know of any disagreement with this plan, if the time seems too long, or of any desire to discontinue therapy. This education is important to all patients regardless of their ethnicity, but particularly so to the Hispanic American, who may be less familiar with psychotherapy.

Physician versus Mental Health Therapist. It is important to explain to the patient not only how mental health therapists differ from general physicians, but also what the similarities are, what a therapist does and does not do. It is important to stress the therapist's potential helpfulness and skills. This explanation is important because Hispanic Americans traditionally tend to go to a family physician even with emotional or psychological problems (Karno, Ross, & Caper, 1969; Padilla *et al.*, 1976).

Self-Evaluation. Each therapist should evaluate his or her own feelings, level of comfort or discomfort, and level of competence in working with Hispanics. If you are uncomfortable as a therapist, you should discuss these feelings with a supervisor or other knowledgeable professionals.

Openness. Encourage the expression of any questions or uncertainties by the patient. Encourage and reward the patient for making specific requests, statements of need, and self-disclosures.

Stress. It is important for the therapist to determine early precisely what the patient's needs are. For example, is the patient coming for help solely with intrapsychic problems, because of external stresses, or for both of these reasons? This point is illustrated by the following case history.

CASE HISTORY

Jorge

Jorge, a Mexican American in his early thirties, came to the clinic voluntarily asking for help. He had never received mental health treatment before.

He was predominantly Spanish-speaking, but recently he had begun studying English. He came into the clinic with problems of hyperventilation, a fear
of choking and dying in his sleep, recurrent anxiety attacks. He was unemployed at the time. He had lived in the United States for about five years,
and before that he had lived in a city in southern Mexico. He had a low self-
image and was experiencing marital difficulties and serious difficulty with
the process of acculturation. Treatment included both a behavioral approach,
to deal with his hyperventilation and anxiety attacks, and a Gestalt therapy
approach, to help him deal with assertiveness, the expression of personal
feelings, his self-image, his difficulties in adapting to a new society, and his
marital difficulties. He also participated in Spanish-speaking group therapy.
While in therapy he was referred to and assisted by a vocational rehabilitation
counselor. In therapy, he showed a great many changes. He stopped the
hyperventilation. His fear of choking and dying and his anxiety attacks virtually disappeared. His self-image improved. He began to speak more clearly
with his wife. With the vocational rehabilitation and his accelerated classes
in English he began to have less difficulty with acculturation.

In this clinical situation, the patient had initially presented with a com
bination of problems, both intrapsychic and environmental, and was able to
receive help for both.

Behavior Therapy

Behavioral approaches may prove very useful in some situations.
For example, a therapist may contract with the patient to target certain
problems and goals or teach the patient specific techniques for relaxation or assertiveness. These approaches may help speed up the
treatment process in some situations by establishing more clearly
defined goals and behaviors. Relaxation training has proven effective
in many situations of anxiety and tension. Assertiveness training may
be a particularly viable approach with patients who have been con-
ditioned to keep their opinions and feelings to themselves. In a comparative study of low-assertive women, for example, Boulette (1976)
found that Hispanic women showed greater gains in assertiveness
and self-esteem through group participation in assertiveness training
than in nondirective psychotherapy.

CASE HISTORY

Alicia and Tony

Alicia, a 26-year-old single Hispanic woman of Costa Rican and Mexican
descent, brought her $3\frac{1}{2}$-year-old son Tony to the clinic for help with his

behavior problems in nursery schools. Alicia did not know where else to turn. She had tried consulting a local *curandero* who had prescribed several prayers and herbs. These did not seem to help. She had also been to her priest, with no changes in Tony's behavior. Alicia stated in the first interview that she was beginning to believe what others were telling her, that perhaps her son had somehow been affected by the devil. The chief complaints about Tony's behavior in school were that he continually disobeyed, disrupted activities, and assaulted other children by hitting them hard, knocking them down, poking them in the eyes, and squeezing them. He had recently been expelled from several nursery schools.

After several home visits, it was evident that Tony was as much of a behavior problem at home as he was in nursery school. It further became clear that his antisocial behavior was being unwittingly reinforced by his family, which consisted of his mother, his uncle, and his grandmother. For example, if he yelled and cried he got what he wanted; he was usually ignored when he was quiet or playing quietly; he was cheered and given much attention when he would fight. Since Tony was not in school at the time of treatment, his behavior problems at home were the treatment focus.

A short-term behavioral therapy program was contracted with Alicia to help change specific behaviors which she considered to be her son's worst. The therapy contract consisted of:

1. Identifying and listing Tony's appropriate behaviors, such as playing calmly with his toys or carrying out a request.
2. Identifying and listing inappropriate behaviors, such as crying to get the television turned on, yelling at her, and hitting other children.
3. Reinforcing appropriate behaviors by hugs, kisses, and other positive regard.
4. Punishing inappropriate behavior by ignoring it or placing him in a room alone for 10-minute time-out periods.
5. Keeping records of the frequency of appropriate and inappropriate behaviors.
6. Reviewing records weekly to assess progress.

The core of this therapy consisted in instructing Alicia on some basic behavioral principles, such as the roles of reward and punishment, modeling, and extinction, and also in instructing and training Alicia to give more positive attention and regard to Tony's appropriate behavior while ignoring his inappropriate behavior. Alicia tried hard and learned quickly. She was encouraged in turn to train her mother and brother on methods of responding to Tony's behavior. She initially met with much open resistance to any changes by her mother but did finally secure good cooperation as her own confidence grew.

A steady decline was seen in most of Tony's antisocial behaviors over an eight-week period. He was obeying Alicia and his grandmother more, he was yelling and crying less as a means to get something, and he seldom hit his grandmother, cousins, or the family cat. His progress continued over an additional four weeks and Alicia reported that her son was behaving like a changed boy. While always loving him, she found herself liking him more and more. Alicia was now receiving compliments for Tony's behavior instead of criticisms.

In a four-month follow-up, Alicia reported that Tony was no problem and was already enrolled in a new nursery school.

In this case, behavioral approaches proved effective in helping a young Hispanic mother and her family successfully realign their responses to her young son who they felt was uncontrollable. It is of further interest that Tony's problem behavior of assaultive hitting of other children in school had been highly reinforced with praise and attention during play-fights with his uncle. It appeared that his rewarded behaviors at home for being *macho*, or manly, had generalized inappropriately to his interactions with other children.

Pharmacological Therapy

Intelligent and judicious use of psychopharmacological interventions can provide effective treatment. However, it has been demonstrated that Hispanic Americans with psychological problems tend to be overmedicated by general practitioners (Acosta, 1977; Karno *et al.*, 1969). Low-income patients also tend to be overmedicated unnecessarily (Hollingshead & Redlich, 1958).

Many of the Spanish-speaking patients seen in public mental health facilities have received minor or major tranquilizers or sedatives for years without adequate diagnostic evaluation or treatment. It is of interest to note that recent findings of Kline, Acosta, Austin, and Johnson (1977) show that both bilingual and Spanish-speaking Mexican-American psychiatric outpatients attribute less importance to psychopharmacological help than do comparative groups of Anglo-American patients. Without question, however, short-term use of medications based on accurate diagnostic assessment can be important if warranted and monitored adequately.

Environmental Intervention

Eclectic therapy with low-income Hispanic Americans has resulted in significant improvement and functioning for many patients. Combined use has been made of the following approaches:

1. An early determination of the patient's expectations, immediate and longer range needs, and recent versus chronic problems.

2. Evaluation of the patient's environmental constraints, degree of acculturation, and problems dealing with referral sources.
3. Use of crisis intervention; determining the most recent crisis and focusing only on the crisis and the goals agreed upon; working within a time frame of up to six sessions.

Now complete the Self-Assessment Exercise 3.3.

SELF-ASSESSMENT EXERCISE 3.3

Discuss the major therapeutic considerations when treating a Hispanic-American patient in a mental health outpatient facility using the following techniques.

1. Psychotherapy

2. Behavior therapy

3. Pharmacological therapy

4. Environmental intervention

When you have completed this exercise, check your answers with those that follow.

SELF-ASSESSMENT EXERCISE 3.3: FEEDBACK

Major therapeutic considerations are as follows:

1. Psychotherapy
   The Hispanic-American patients will require substantial expressions of friendliness and encouragement to discuss their feelings and problems and express any disagreements with their therapists. They should be given adequate instruction about the nature of psychotherapy and they should participate directly in defining the therapeutic plan. Careful consideration should be given to both emotional problems and problems of living.

2. Behavior therapy
   Behavior modification techniques such as assertiveness training and relaxation training have characteristics which fit very closely Hispanic Americans' preconceptions about therapy, for example, short time period, specific goals, and immediate reward for accomplishments.

3. Pharmacological therapy
   There seems to be a tendency for therapists to select medication as the treatment of choice with the Hispanic-American patient. Although this mode of treatment is a valuable therapeutic tool, adequate care must be exercised in diagnosing the patient's problem, choosing the medication, and monitoring its effectiveness.

4. Environmental intervention
   The problems of living which are faced by the typical Hispanic-American patient often require active intervention on the part of the therapist. In order to do this, the therapist must be aware of the patient's special problems, know about appropriate community resources, and be determined to handle the patient's double neediness.

If your answers correspond closely with those above, please continue reading. If not, please reread the preceding material.

SUMMARY

Hispanic Americans represent a substantial proportion of the patients coming to a mental health outpatient clinic for treatment. They have unique problems caused by the need to use two different languages, the reconciliation of two different cultural beliefs, low economic and educational resources, as well as lack of knowledge about community service resources available to assist them.

In the therapy situation therapists must make a special effort to correctly diagnose patients' emotional problems as well as their problems of living. Only then can appropriate therapeutic interventions be effectively applied.

REFERENCES

Acosta, F. X. Ethnic variables in psychotherapy: The Mexican American. In J. L. Martinez (Ed.), *Chicano psychology*. New York: Academic Press, 1977.

Acosta, F. X. Barriers between mental health services and Mexican Americans: An examination of a paradox. *American Journal of Community Psychology*, 1979, 7, 503–520.

Acosta, F. X., & Cristo, M. H. Development of a bilingual interpreter program: An alternative model for Spanish-speaking services. *Professional Psychology*, 1981, 12, 474–482.

Acosta, F. X., & Sheehan, J. G. Preferences toward Mexican American and Anglo American psychotherapists. *Journal of Consulting and Clinical Psychology*, 1976, 44, 272–279.

Boulette, T. R. Assertive training with low-income Mexican American women. In M. R. Miranda (Ed.), *Psychotherapy with the Spanish-speaking: Issues in research and service delivery*. Los Angeles: Spanish Speaking Mental Health Research Center, University of California, 1976.

Casavantes, E. *El Tecato*. Washington, D.C.: Coalition of Spanish Speaking Mental Health and Health Organizations, 1975.

Dworkin, A. G. Stereotypes and self-images held by native-born and foreign-born Mexican Americans. *Sociology and Social Research*, 1965, 49, 214–224.

Edgarton, R. B., Karno, M., & Fernandez, I. *Curanderismo* in the metropolis. *American Journal of Psychotherapy*, 1970, 24, 124–134.

Fabrega, H., & Wallace, C. A. Value identification and psychiatric disability: An analysis involving Americans of Mexican descent. *Behavior Science*, 1968, 13, 362–371

Grebler, L., Moore, J. W., & Guzman, R. C. *The Mexican-American people. The nation's second largest minority*. New York: Free Press, 1970.

Heiman, E. M., Burruel, G., & Chavez, N. Factors determining effective psychiatric outpatient treatment for Mexican Americans. *Hospital and Community Psychiatry*, 1975, 26, 515–517.

Hernandez, J., Estrada, L., & Alvirez, D. Census data and the problem of conceptually defining the Mexican American population. *Social Science Quarterly*, 1973, 53, 671–687.

Hollingshead, A. B., & Redlich, F. C. *Social class and mental illness: A community study*. New York: Wiley, 1958.

Kagan, S., & Buriel, R. Field dependence–independence and Mexican-American culture and education. In J. L. Martinez (Ed.), *Chicano psychology*. New York: Academic Press, 1977.

Karno, M. The enigma of ethnicity in a psychiatric clinic. *Archives of General Psychiatry*, 1966, 14, 516–520.

Karno, M., & Edgarton, R. B. Perception of mental illness in a Mexican-American community. *Archives of General Psychiatry*, 1969, 20, 233–238.

Karno, M., & Morales, A. A community mental health service for Mexican Americans in a metropolis. *Comprehensive Psychiatry*, 1971, 12, 116–121.

Karno, M., Ross, R. N., & Caper, R. A. Mental health roles of physicians in a Mexican-American community. *Community Mental Health Journal*, 1969, *5*, 62–69.

Kiev, A. *Curanderismo: Mexican-American folk psychiatry.* New York: Free Press, 1968.

Kline, F., Acosta, F. X., Austin, W., & Johnson, R. G. Subtle bias in the treatment of the Spanish speaking patient. In E. R. Padilla and A. M. Padilla (Eds.), *Transcultural psychiatry: An Hispanic perspective.* Los Angeles: Spanish Speaking Mental Health Research Center, University of California, 1977.

Kline, F., Acosta, F. X., Austin, W., & Johnson, R. G. The misunderstood Spanish-speaking patient. *American Journal of Psychiatry*, 1980, *137*, 1530–1533.

LeVine, E. S., & Padilla, A. M. *Crossing cultures in therapy pluralistic counseling for the Hispanic.* Monterey, Calif.: Brooks/Cole, 1980.

Los Angeles County. Population report Los Angeles County. (Evaluation, Research & Statistics report NO. F-640). Los Angeles: County of Los Angeles Department of Health Services, 1978.

Marcos, L. R., & Alpert, M. Strategies and risks in psychotherapy with bilingual patients: The phenomenon of language independence. *American Journal of Psychiatry*, 1976, *133*, 1275–1278.

Murillo, N. The Mexican-American family. In C. A. Hernandez, M. J. Haug, & N. N. Wagner (Eds.), *Chicanos: Social and psychological perspectives* (2nd ed.). Saint Louis: C. V. Mosby, 1971.

Padilla, A. M., Carlos, M. L., & Keefe, S. E. Mental health service utilization by Mexican Americans. In M. R. Miranda (Ed.), *Psychotherapy with the Spanish-speaking: Issues in research and service delivery.* Los Angeles: Spanish Speaking Mental Health Research Center, University of California, 1976.

Padilla, A. M., Ruiz, R. A., & Alvarez, R. A. Community mental health services for the Spanish-speaking/surnamed population. *American Psychologist*, 1975, *30*, 892–905.

Penalosa, F. Mexican family roles. *Journal of Marriage and the Family*, 1968, *30*, 680–689.

President's Commission on Mental Health. *Report to the President* (Vol. 1). Washington, D.C.: U.S. Government Printing Office, 1978.

Russell, G., & Satterwhite, B. It's your turn in the sun. *Time*, October 16, 1978, pp. 48–61.

Srole, L., Langer, T. S., Michael, S. T., Opler, M. K., & Rennie, T. A. C. *Mental health in the metropolis: The Midtown Manhattan study.* New York: McGraw-Hill, 1962.

Stonequist, E. V. *The marginal man: A study in personality and culture conflict.* New York: Russell & Russell, 1961.

Sue, S. Community mental health services to minority groups: Some optimism, some pessimism. *American Psychologist*, 1977, *32*, 616–624.

U.S. Bureau of Census. *Statistical abstract of the United States: 1974* (95th ed.). Washington, D.C.: U.S. Government Printing Office, 1974.

U.S. Bureau of the Census. *Statistical abstract of the United States: 1980 (101st edition).* Washington, D.C.: U.S. Government Printing Office, 1980.

Velasquez de la Cadena, M., Gray, E., & Iribas, J. L. *Velasquez Spanish and English Dictionary,* Chicago: Follett, 1974.

Yamamoto, J., James, Q. C., Bloombaum, M., & Hattem, J. Racial factors in patient selection. *American Journal of Psychiatry*, 1967, *124*, 630–636.

CHAPTER 4

The Black American Patient

Barbara A. Bass, Frank X. Acosta, and Leonard A. Evans

INTRODUCTION

Important sociocultural factors in the psychological evaluation and treatment of black American patients are often overlooked or misinterpreted by psychotherapists. This situation stems from two primary sources: the therapist's paucity of information regarding similarities and differences between the dominant culture and that of the black American, and myths about black Americans that result from misinformation obtained from scientific inquiries of questionable validity as reported in the literature.

The lack of importance attached to knowledge of black American culture can be assessed by reviewing the indexes of the main textbooks currently used in psychiatric training institutions. No reference to "Negro," "black," "race," or "racism" is to be found in Noyes and Kolb's *Modern Clinical Psychiatry* (1968), Freedman and Kaplan's first edition of *The Comprehensive Textbook of Psychiatry* (1967), or in Alexander and Selesnick's *The History of Psychiatry* (1966). Revised editions of Freedman and Kaplan (1975) and of Kolb (1977) do contain passing references to these items.

Closely associated with the deficiencies in the instructional literature is an absence of formal training in the psychiatric evaluation and treatment of black American patients. The course catalogs of 10 prominent American medical schools were reviewed, and none contained descriptions which appear to address themselves to this issue (Wyatt, Bass, & Powell, 1978). Further, other mental health disciplines seldom, if ever, include specific training relevant to the treatment of black Americans (President's Commission on Mental Health, 1978).

Social science research on black Americans typically attempts to point out why there are individual, family, and community deficits among black Americans. Such research is thus often not free from bias. It is difficult to understand the life-styles of black Americans using traditional theories and procedures, which were actually developed by white behavioral and social scientists to explain the behavior of white Americans. When these criteria are applied to the black American, the data may indicate various deficits, and inferiority-oriented conclusions may then be drawn.

After completing this chapter and a corresponding group discussion session, the reader should be able to:

1. Describe the sociocultural characteristics of black Americans which may affect the service they receive at a mental health facility
2. Describe the important attitudes of the black American toward mental health services
3. Discuss the most common problems faced by therapists when treating black American patients
4. Describe and use therapeutic approaches which are most effective with black American patients
5. Express satisfaction with the process and outcome of therapeutic encounters with the black American patient

Please read the above learning objectives until you become familiar with the goals of this chapter, then continue reading.

CHARACTERISTICS OF THE BLACK AMERICAN

Diversity of Life-Style

Black American culture has been observed and described in a variety of ways. Blacks are often termed culturally deprived or disadvantaged, culturally deficient or different, underprivileged, or socially deprived. Such terms have led many social and behavioral scientists to believe that black Americans as a group are culturally deprived and psychologically maladjusted. They suggest that when compared to that of white Americans, the environment in which black Americans were reared as children, and in which they continue to rear their own children, lacks the necessary early experiences to prepare them for excellence in school, appropriate sex-role behavior, and economic achievement (Bernstein, 1960; Hunt, 1971; Lewis, 1966; Moynihan, 1965; Riessman, 1962). In short, black American people are sometimes perceived as culturally and psychologically deprived because their experiential background provides inferior preparation for effective movement within the dominant white culture.

Unfortunately, this negative conceptualization of black American culture may result from a lack of valid research. Currently, there is only a limited understanding of the variety of black American life-styles that exist in the United States. This limitation results in a tendency to generalize and to assume that there is a singular black American life-style that is different and inferior to the white American life-style.

Recently black American social scientists such as Billingsley (1968) and Hill (1972) have attempted to correct these negative generalizations by studying the diversity of life-styles in the black American community. Hill, for example, identifies and analyzes five characteristics or strengths which lead toward survival, advancement, and stability of black American families: adaptability of family roles, strong kinship bonds, strong work orientation, strong achievement orientation, and strong religious orientation. It is interesting that these characteristics are very similar to those needed for achievement in the white community.

Billingsley suggests that black Americans represent an ethnic subsociety which, like other ethnic subsocieties, may be broken down into three social dimensions: social class, rural or urban residence, and region of the country lived in.

Social Status: Equitable or Inequitable

The most recent evidence (U.S. Department of Commerce, 1979) indicates that blacks are represented in the upper, middle, and lower classes, despite the phenomenon that more has been written about the black lower class.

A major problem encountered when describing the social class among black Americans is that the criteria developed by social scientists, namely, education and occupation, are generally more reliable in categorizing whites than blacks. For example, white school principals and their families are considered middle class. However, in all probability black school principals would be considered upper class by the black community (Billingsley, 1968). Factors such as respectability and community activity are highly valued in the black community, along with education and occupation.

An additional striking problem often noted in population reports (e.g., Smythe & Smythe, 1976) is that black Americans typically do not receive the same return for their education as do white Americans across all classes. More specifically, blacks with education comparable to whites do not have the same occupational opportunities, and for those with comparable occupations, they do not receive the same incomes (Langer, Gersten, Green, Eisenberg, Herson, & McCarthy, 1974).

In family studies, for example, it has been shown that within any range of incomes black families will cluster toward the lower end of the range and white families toward the upper end (Billingsley, 1968). For black families to maintain middle-class status, at least two persons must be employed, and therefore extended family members must be available to help care for the children.

The report of the Joint Commission on Mental Health of Children (1970) concluded that there is a very strong relationship between poverty and minority-group status. The report noted that unemployment, underemployment, and low wages are more prevalent among minority groups; that education does not always provide upward mobility for minorities as it does for the majority; and that "among the multiple causes of poverty are racist policies and attitudes."

The intent here is not to deny the many problems that black Americans face in white society but rather to show that the economic, political, and social forces of the larger society strongly affect the conditions which determine black life-styles.

Social Class Life-Styles

About 10% of black families constitute the upper echelon of the black community. These are the families whose heads of household are highly educated, often with graduate degrees, who are in the higher income levels, who have secure occupations in which advancement is possible, and who live in comfortable housing (Billingsley, 1968).

If these same additional variables are considered, black American middle class families account for about 40% of all black families. Within this group, however, there are three distinct subgroupings: upper middle class, solid middle class, and precarious middle class. These are distinguished by educational, income, and occupational achievement, and by the security of their hold on middle-class status.

Finally, there are the lower classes, where about 50% of all black American families are located. Again, however, there are several groupings, which may be distinguished by the education, income, and occupational history and security of the head of the respective families: the working nonpoor, the working poor, and the nonworking poor. The first group, the working nonpoor, is comprised of semiskilled workers who have a stable and secure niche in unionized industry. The largest group, the working poor, consists of unskilled and service workers with marginal incomes. The final group, the nonworking poor, is the one about which most information appears in the literature and public press. Comprising about one-quarter of all lower-class black families, it consists of those who are unemployed or intermittently employed and supported by relatives and friends or by public welfare (Billingsley, 1968).

Some lower-class black families live a middle-class life-style, placing emphasis upon decorous public behavior and general respectability, insisting that their children "get an education" and "make something of themselves." They prize family stability, and an unwed mother is something much more serious than "just a girl who had an accident"; premarital and extramarital relationships, if indulged in at all, must be discreet. For this type of family, social life is organized around churches, volunteer associations of all types, and, for women, "the cult of clothes" is so important that fashion shows are a popular fund-raising activity even in churches. For both men and women, owning a home and going into business are highly desired goals, the former recently becoming a more realistic one, the latter a mere fantasy. Today, home ownership is even more difficult to achieve due to higher interest mortgage rates.

Within the same income range, and not always at the lower margin of it, other black American families live an "organized lower-class life style." The "organized" lower class is oriented primarily around churches whose preachers, often semiliterate, exhort them to "be in the 'world' but not of it." Conventional middle-class morality is preached, although a general attitude of "the spirit is willing, but the flesh is weak" prevails except among a minority fully committed to the Pentecostal sects (Drake, 1970).

In the organized lower class, young people with talent find wide scope for expressing it in choirs, quartets, and so on, which travel from church to church and sometimes from city to city. Adults as well as young people find satisfaction and, indeed, prestige in serving as ushers and deacons, "mothers," Sunday school teachers, and choir leaders.

At the lowest income levels, an "unorganized" lower-class lifestyle exists; members tend to be involved in gambling, excessive drinking, narcotics, and sexual promiscuity. For this group, violent interpersonal relations reflect an ethos of suspicion and resentment. It is within this milieu that criminal and semicriminal activities burgeon (Drake, 1970).

Valentine (1968) stresses the need to distinguish between cultural values and situational or circumstantial adaptations. It is a misconception that people live the way they do because they prefer their actual mode of existence and its consequences. In a highly stratified social system like that of the United States, poor people have a narrow margin of choice as to how they live. It is risky to infer a group's preferences and potentialities from adaptations forced upon them by their conditions of existence (Ryan, 1971).

Self-Identity and Skin Color

Spurlock (1973) has shown that black children who felt most secure about themselves identified with being black. Those who felt the least secure made more of an out-group identification and also had more hostility toward whites.

Spurlock also notes that although some black American children proclaim "black is beautiful," they may still harbor negative feelings about their racial identity. This is particularly characteristic among children from lower socioeconomic groups, who may be exposed to more discriminatory and rejecting experiences than those from more sheltered backgrounds. Skin color is an important issue here because the darker the skin the more problems one encounters.

Community Network

Black American families place heavy emphasis and reliance on interactions with both relatives and nonrelatives. Therefore, people of importance in the community—elders, ministers, teachers, or other responsible adults—have always been called upon to help the family socialize its children. Many black Americans can point to a member of the community who made the difference between success and failure.

There are several ways in which community members supplement the efforts of the family. They may serve as extensions of the parents and may instruct, discipline, assist, and otherwise guide the young of a given family. They may serve as role models and show an interest in the young people. As advocates, they may actively intercede with major segments of society to help young black Americans find opportunities which might otherwise have been closed to them. As supportive figures, they may simply inquire about the progress of the young and take a special interest in them. In more formal roles, such as teacher or elder, community members are more readily able to serve youth as a part of their general occupation.

Now complete the Self-Assessment Exercise 4.1.

SELF-ASSESSMENT EXERCISE 4.1

1. Discuss the diversity of life-styles which are represented by black American families.

2. Describe the characteristics of black American families which fall within the following social categories.

    a. Upper class

    b. Middle class

    c. Lower class

3. Discuss the relationship between skin color and childhood attitudes.

4. Discuss the importance of the community network to the black American.

When you have completed this exercise, check your answers with those that follow.

SELF-ASSESSMENT EXERCISE 4.1: FEEDBACK

1. Contrary to the scientific literature, which focuses on the lower class, there are three distinct classes and a variety of life-styles among black Americans. As Billingsley points out, members within an ethnic group vary on three social dimensions: social class, urban or rural residence, and region of the country lived in.

2. The characteristics of black families which fall within the following social categories are as follows:

   a. Upper class: Comprises approximately 10% of all blacks; the family heads are highly educated, in the high income levels, have secure occupations, and provide comfortable housing.
   b. Middle class: Approximately 40% of all black families may be considered middle class. Three distinct groupings can be found: upper, solid, and precarious middle class. They are distinguished by education, income, and occupational achievement, and by the security of their hold on middle-class status.
   c. Lower class: Approximately half of all black American families are located in the lower class and fall into three groups: working nonpoor, working poor, and nonworking poor. They are distinguished by occupational history, job security of their heads, education, and income.

3. Children who feel most secure about themselves identified with being black. Those who feel least secure make more of an out-group identification and also have more hostility toward whites.

4. Black Americans place great importance and receive considerable support from relatives and people of importance in the community. Therapists should weave their treatment around the patient's community network.

If your answers correspond closely with those above, please continue reading. If not, please reread the preceding material.

ATTITUDES TOWARD MENTAL HEALTH SERVICES

According to the President's Commission on Mental Health (1978), an increasing number of black American families from widely divergent cultural, economic, and experiential backgrounds are seeking mental health services. This is a significant change in the attitude and behavior of blacks as reported in 1960 by Gurin, Veroff, and Feld.

Gurin *et al.* suggested that black Americans feared psychotherapy or mental health services because the need for such services was viewed as an indication of weakness or severe mental problems requiring hospitalization. Despite the increase in the number of blacks using mental health services, the commission's report indicates that significant inequities exist in the availability of services, the quality of care, and the types of treatment offered to black Americans and other minority groups. Compared to whites, blacks are significantly less often the recipients of individual or group psychotherapy; they spend less time in the hospital; and they are often discharged without referral (Mayo, 1974).

When ethnic differences are accompanied by low socioeconomic status, there are decided differences in types and duration of treatment (Yamamoto, James, Bloombaum, & Hattem, 1967). In Langer *et al.*'s (1974) study in Manhattan, it was found that therapy was not "wasted" on black Americans or Spanish-speaking children. For example, black Americans were referred to school counselors and sometimes to a social worker; Spanish-speaking children were less often referred to either. The white children were more likely to be referred to a psychiatrist regardless of income. According to the commission report, the delivery of mental health services to minority group children is beset with many obstacles, including: (1) maldistribution of mental health professionals; (2) attitudinal barriers; (3) lack of coordination among agencies; (4) lack of continuity of care; (5) lack of access to services; and (6) problems of communication and emphasis.

It has been shown that blacks in need of psychological help will avoid mental health services because of a basic mistrust of white therapists (Comer, 1973; Jackson, 1973). The implication here is that blacks would favor psychotherapy if more black therapists were available.

Some empirical support for the above position is found in the recent work of Wolkon, Moriwaki, and Williams (1973). Wolkon *et al.* found that black college females significantly preferred black therapists, whereas white college females showed no racial preference. In addition, black lower-class subjects were found to hold more negative attitudes toward psychotherapy than either black or white middle-class subjects. Although these findings suggest that blacks may have preferences for black therapists and may profit more in therapy through a racial match, they further indicate that one's class may be more important than race in attitudes toward therapy.

Vontress (1970) states that black males provide greater difficulty to counselors than black females. This is interpreted as indicating that blacks generally disclose less about themselves than whites, and that black males disclose less than females (Jourard & Lasakow, 1958).

On the other hand, other investigators contend that the problem of blacks receiving inadequate mental health services relative to their needs may not exist so much in their pretherapy attitudes but in the kind of services they receive (Acosta, 1980; Sue, McKinney, Allen, & Hall, 1974; Thomas & Sillen, 1972). In a recent interview study with low-income men and women who had prematurely terminated from therapy after two sessions in a public psychiatric outpatient clinic, Acosta found an intriguing contrast in the responses of black patients. The primary reason given by these patients for their early self-termination was a negative attitude toward the therapist. The majority of the therapists were white and of middle-class backgrounds. In spite of their negative attitude, however, black patients still reported a moderately positive attitude toward the potential usefulness of counseling and therapy for themselves and others in the future. The implication here was that while the black patients may have expressed negative feelings about their brief therapy experiences, they were still willing to see therapy as a possible resource if needed in the future.

Sue et al. (1974) further reported the importance of existing community mental health facilities to blacks as evidenced by a high rate of use. In the Seattle, Washington, area blacks utilize facilities at a higher rate proportionate to their population. However, major problems were identified in the services received by blacks. For example, there was a disproportionate use of paraprofessional staff at the intake session during therapy. In addition, over half of the black clients dropped out of therapy after the first session. The exact reasons are not known.

A high rate of black utilization was also found for outpatient mental health services in Los Angeles, California (Los Angeles County, 1973, 1975). Admission rates show an increase from 19.4% of total admissions in 1970 to 26.1% in 1974, although only 12% of the population is black.

These utilization figures underscore the fact that black Americans are at least applying for initial visits at mental health facilities in increasing numbers and at much higher rates than expected. These facts suggest that there is a generally favorable attitude toward the use of mental health services within the black American community.

Now complete the Self-Assessment Exercise 4.2.

SELF-ASSESSMENT EXERCISE 4.2

Describe the factors which affect the attitude of black Americans toward mental health services.

When you have completed this exercise, check your answer with the one that follows.

SELF-ASSESSMENT EXERCISE 4.2: FEEDBACK

The attitude of black Americans toward mental health services can be inferred from the fact that increasing numbers of them are seeking such services. This suggests that there is a generally favorable attitude toward the use of mental health services. However, problems that arise in the delivery of services may be more closely related to the patient's social class and to the therapist's race. Black patients have encountered difficulties in receiving a full range of mental health services and often leave these services prematurely.

If your answers correspond closely with those above, please continue reading. If not, please reread the preceding material.

PROBLEMS IN TREATING BLACK AMERICAN PATIENTS

Social Support System

The social support systems used by black Americans are often misinterpreted by white therapists. The need for them is seen by some white therapists as a weakness in the patient's personality. For example, patients' desire to involve extended family members and significant others in their treatment has often been viewed by therapists as a form of resistance and overdependence on the part of the patient (Wyatt, Reardon, & Bass, 1977). Contrary to this view, failure of the therapist to involve significant others in the therapy of the patient, when appropriate and available, can lead to alienation of the patient. Such an error or oversight, more often than not, is caused by resistance on the part of the therapist to becoming intimately involved in the therapy of the patient.

Cultural Factors

The therapist's lack of understanding, acknowledgment, and appreciation of sociocultural factors can also represent a form of resistance. Therapists, when taken out of the role of being the expert, may become reluctant to ask their patients to explain or clarify certain aspects of their culture such as values, roles, language, and behavior. For example, a therapist may believe the stereotype that black people are never on time for appointments. As a result, the therapist may not ask why the patient arrived late for an appointment. It is possible that the patient is late because of resistance or some reluctance to come in, economic reasons, lack of transportation, or lack of awareness that the sessions are expected to begin at the appointed time. Therapists cannot know the reasons unless they ask.

Communication Style

There are also differences in communication style that can be misinterpreted by the therapist. For some black Americans, initial mistrust is often expressed by avoiding direct eye contact, giving limited answers to questions, or providing few details. Such behavior may also be due to past sociocultural conditioning or a preference for physical action rather than verbal expression. This rather abrupt behavior is often interpreted by the therapist as a lack of insight and poor verbal skills. In order to counteract this tendency on the part of patients, therapists may need to explain the role expectations of therapist and patient within the psychotherapeutic setting. In addition, therapists may need to be more sensitive to developing patient trust and putting them at ease. This would be particularly important with those who have no prior experience in mental health treatment and who may assume that therapists function like medical doctors: they ask questions and give advice.

Skin Color

Skin color differentially affects the experience, culture, and psychology of black Americans. To ignore the formative influence of these differences in history and social existence is an error. It is very important for white therapists who have a working knowledge of black culture to discuss with their patients the possible effects of skin color on their interpersonal communication.

However, a primary drawback to this approach is that few white middle-class therapists have adequate information concerning patients of different racial or ethnic origins. For example, the American Psychoanalytic Society reports that 99% of the patients of white psychoanalysts in this country are white. Therefore, therapists frequently lack understanding of the possible effects of skin color differences on the effectiveness of psychotherapy.

If a therapist is uncomfortable talking with a patient about racial differences, it may indicate resistance to therapeutic involvement. If a therapist has such blind spots, it may cause difficulties if the patient begins to discuss that particular issue.

To view racial differences as just one of several potential barriers to effective psychotherapy, and not a very special one, would be an error. Usually the issue of race comes up in the first few weeks, often in the first hour of psychotherapy. If the patient hasn't brought it up in the first session, some therapists bring it up themselves. It is often most helpful to discuss this issue because of its potential effects upon the effectiveness of psychotherapy.

Minority Practice

Some therapists are reluctant to see minority patients because they do not want their private practice to be labeled as a minority practice. It is not uncommon for therapists to make negative comments about the number of minority patients seen by their few colleagues who do treat minority patients. Many therapists are unable to deal with their own prejudices and therefore are critical of colleagues who can.

Patient Referrals

An additional problem may arise if a patient is referred for psychotherapy and the information you receive is based upon culturally biased testing, inadequate history taking, lack of understanding, or misinterpretation of the patient's culture and behavior. It will be the therapist's responsibility to assess the quality of such information and respond appropriately.

Black Dialect

A subtle problem in interracial psychotherapy is demonstrated in verbal behavior. For example, a patient may "jive" (clown or trick) the therapist through the use of language. The language commonly used is that of the patient's peer group. The therapist may be entertained by this but may not be aware that it could represent very subtle resistance on the part of the patient.

Jive talk has several purposes. On the one hand, black dialect may represent the only mode of verbal communication available to the patient and may allow for the expression of feelings that otherwise may be isolated out of the therapy. On the other hand, jive talk may serve to block the expression of some of the patient's inner feelings. The therapist must be sensitive to the patient's cues and use of jive language. For example, jive may be used to maintain distance with the therapist; it may be a manifestation of past relationships with other whites inappropriately acted out with the therapist. The patient may lapse into black dialect and have to interpret for the therapist unless he wants to keep the therapist out, in which case the therapist should recognize that there is a barrier and help the patient deal with the resistance.

Discrimination

The preponderance of evidence clearly indicates that a person's social class is important in determining whether or not he or she will be offered treatment. In addition, social class may often determine the assigned therapist's level of training and experience (Jones, 1974; Sue, 1977). As we have indicated before, Hollingshead and Redlich (1958) argue that psychiatrists tend to select "good" patients, that is, those who possess social and intellectual standards similar to their own. Rosenthal and Frank (1958) similarly conclude that "psychiatrists considered as good candidates for psychotherapy those patients with whom they can more easily communicate and who share their value systems." Schofield (1964) refers to these as the YAVIS patients,—young, attractive, verbal, intelligent, and successful.

It could be argued that therapists' low evaluation of black American clients may be related to the assumption that all or most of them are lower class. Thomas and Sillen (1972) strongly assert that black stereotypes abound among therapists and parallel those of American society in general. Table 4.1 which follows suggests such a parallel.

Individualized Treatment

It is very important to understand that there is not just one therapeutic orientation that can be considered the only approach in

Table 4.1. Attitudes of American Society and
Mental Health Professionals toward Blacks[a]

American society	Mental health professionals
Lazy	Unmotivated
Unintelligent	Unintelligent (no introspective thinking, concrete, lack of insight, nonverbal)
Unhealthy	Not psychologically minded, higher incidence of psychiatric disorders
Criminal	Impulse ridden; mistrustful
Sexual	Primitive characteristics

[a] This table is reconstructed from material in Thomas and Sillen (1972).

the treatment of black Americans. However, it is essential that the therapist establish a trusting patient–therapist relationship.

It is hoped that a well-trained, sensitive, and knowledgeable therapist—despite his or her particular theoretical frame of reference or the patient's ethnicity—will determine on an *individual basis* the patient's needs and the therapeutic approach that most effectively meets those needs. For example, a patient who is in crisis will need crisis intervention until the crisis is resolved; any other form of psychotherapeutic intervention at this time would be futile.

Now please complete the Self-Assessment Exercise 4.3.

SELF-ASSESSMENT EXERCISE 4.3

Discuss sociocultural factors which therapists need to be aware of in each of the following categories:

a. Social support systems

b. Cultural factors

c. Communication style

d. Skin color

e. Minority practice

f. Patient referrals

g. Black dialect

h. Discrimination

i. Individualized treatment

When you have completed this exercise, check your answers with those that follow.

SELF-ASSESSMENT EXERCISE 4.3: FEEDBACK

The sociocultural factors and issues about which therapists need to be aware within each of the following categories are as follows.

a. Social support systems

For many black Americans, extended family members and other significant persons within their environment provide emotional and psychological support. The inclusion of such persons in psychiatric assessment and treatment may provide the therapist with valuable information and understanding regarding the patient's family life, interpersonal relationships, and available supports that may be helpful to the patient in dealing with what can often be a hostile environment.

b. Cultural factors

Any differences between the patient and therapist regarding life-styles, values, roles, language, and behavior should be openly acknowledged and discussed in the therapeutic relationship to insure correct interpretations and better understanding.

c. Communication style

For any patient new to psychotherapy, initial mistrust or anxiety may be expressed through lack of eye contact or other nonverbal communication. The therapist must ask questions of the patient and explain the therapeutic process to avoid misinterpretation of the behavior.

d. Skin color

Historically, skin color in our society has been an important issue and has led to discrimination against black Americans. Therapists need to acknowledge the issue of skin color in therapy and be aware of their own and their patients' feelings about racial differences.

e. Minority practice

The majority of psychotherapists in private practice see few minority patients either because they don't want their practice to be labeled a "minority practice" or because they may be uncomfortable in dealing with their own prejudices.

f. Patient referrals

Patients may be referred who have been diagnosed according to standardized tests which may be culturally biased. The therapist has the responsibility of knowing the uses and abuses of psychological testing in order to assess the quality and validity of such information.

g. Black dialect

Jive talk serves several purposes. On the one hand, black dialect may allow for the expression of feelings that otherwise may be isolated out of the therapy.

On the other hand, jive talk may serve to block the expression of some of the patient's inner feelings. The therapist must be sensitive to the patient's cues and use of jive language.

h. Discrimination
The stereotypes and attitudes held by society about blacks may also be held by psychotherapists and will affect the delivery, the length, and the type of services received. Therapists tend to select patients with whom they are most comfortable and who are most similar to themselves.

i. Individualized treatment
In selecting treatment strategies for patients, the primary consideration is the patients' needs—not ethnicity. There is no single therapeutic approach for a particular ethnic group. It is the responsibility of therapists to receive good training in various therapeutic approaches and to select from their repertoire the approach that seems most appropriate to the needs of the individual patient. The therapist should keep in mind the sociocultural factors and the problems faced by black Americans in this society, as well as their effects on the particular patient, and acknowledge these issues in the treatment provided.

If your answers correspond closely with those above, please continue reading. If not, please reread the preceding material.

SUMMARY

In order to judge what is healthy or disturbed in an individual's psychological functioning, a therapist must be aware of what is appropriate and effective within the patient's specific cultural milieu. For mental health professionals involved with patients whose cultural and experiential backgrounds may differ from theirs, this becomes crucial to the delivery of effective mental health services.

Information concerning sociocultural factors that may be important in the diagnosis and treatment of minority patients is often omitted from traditional professional education. In spite of this lack, the mental health professional must know and understand sociocultural variables in order to provide the most effective psychotherapeutic approach for the black American patient. Additional educational programs in this area are critically needed.

The most effective therapeutic approach for an individual is one which is tailored to the specific needs of that individual. There is not a single "most effective therapeutic approach" for black American patients.

REFERENCES

Acosta, F. X. Self-described reasons for premature termination of psychotherapy by Mexican American, Black American, and Anglo-American patients. *Psychological Reports*, 1980, *47*, 435–443.

Alexander, F. G., & Selesnick, S. T. *The history of psychiatry*. New York: Harper & Row, 1966.

Bernstein, B. Language and social class. *British Journal of Sociology*, 1960, *2*, 271–276.

Billingsley, A. *Black families in white America*. Englewood Cliffs, N.J.: Prentice-Hall, 1968.

Comer, J. P. The need is now. *Mental Health*, 1973, *57*, 3–6.

Drake, S. C. The social and economic status of the Negro in the United States. In R. Endo & W. Strawbridge (Eds.), *Perspectives on black America*. Englewood Cliffs, N.J.: Prentice-Hall, 1970.

Freedman, A. M., & Kaplan, H. I. *The comprehensive textbook of psychiatry* (1st ed.). Baltimore: Williams & Wilkins, 1967.

Freedman, A. M., & Kaplan, H. I. *The comprehensive textbook of psychiatry* (2nd ed.). Baltimore: Williams & Wilkins, 1975.

Gurin, G., Veroff, J., & Feld, S. *Americans view their mental health*. New York: Basic Books, 1960.

Hill, R. *The strengths of black families: A National Urban League research study*. New York: Emerson Hall, 1972.

Hollingshead, A. B., & Redlich, F. C. *Social class and mental illness: A community study*. New York: Wiley, 1958.

Hunt, J. M. Parent and child centers: Their basis in the behavioral and educational sciences. *American Journal of Orthopsychiatry*, 1971, *41*, 13–42.

Jackson, A. Psychotherapy: Factors associated with the race of the therapist. *Psychotherapy: Theory, Research and Practice*, 1973, *10*, 273–277.

Joint Commission on Mental Health of Children. *Crises in child mental health*. New York: Harper & Row, 1970.

Jones, E. Social class and psychotherapy: A critical review of research. *Psychiatry*, 1974, *37*, 307–320.

Jourard, S. M., & Lasakow, P. Some factors in self-disclosure. *Journal of Abnormal and Social Psychology*, 1958, *56*, 91–98.

Kolb, L. C. *Modern clinical psychiatry* (9th ed.). Philadelphia: Saunders, 1977.

Langer, T. S., Gersten, J., Green, E. I., Eisenberg, J. G., Herson, J. J., & McCarthy, E. D. Treatment of psychological disorders among urban children. *Journal of Consulting and Clinical Psychology*, 1974, *42*, 170–179.

Lewis, O. The culture of poverty. *Scientific American*, 1966, *215*, 19–25.

Los Angeles County. *Patient and Service Statistics* (Report No. 10). Los Angeles: County of Los Angeles Department of Health Services, Mental Health Services, 1973.

Los Angeles County. *Patient and Service Statistics* (Report No. 11). Los Angeles: County of Los Angeles Department of Health Services, Mental Health Services, 1975.

Mayo, J. A. The significance of sociocultural variables in the psychiatric treatment of black outpatients. *Comprehensive Psychiatry*, 1974, *15*, 471–482.

Moynihan, D. P. *The Negro family: A case for national action.* Washington, D.C.: U.S. Department of Labor, Office of Policy Planning and Research, March 1965.

Noyes, A. P., & Kolb, L. C. *Modern clinical psychiatry* (7th ed.). Philadelphia: Saunders, 1968.

President's Commission on Mental Health. *Report to the President* (Vol. 1). Washington, D.C.: U.S. Government Printing Office, 1978.

Riessman, F. *The culturally deprived child.* New York: Harper & Row, 1962.

Rosenthal, D., & Frank, J. D. The fate of psychiatric clinic outpatients assigned to psychotherapy. *Journal of Nervous and Mental Disease,* 1958, *127,* 330–343.

Ryan, W. *Blaming the victim.* New York: Pantheon, 1971.

Schofield, W. *Psychotherapy: The purchase of friendship.* Englewood Cliffs, N.J.: Prentice-Hall, 1964.

Smythe, M., & Smythe, H. *Black-American reference book.* Englewood Cliffs, N.J.: Prentice-Hall, 1976.

Spurlock, J. Some consequences of racism for children. In C. V. Willie, B. M. Kramer, & B. S. Brown (Eds.), *Racism and mental health essay.* Pittsburgh: University of Pittsburgh Press, 1973.

Sue, S. Community mental health services to minority groups: Some optimism, some pessimism. *American Psychologist,* 1977, *32,* 616–624.

Sue, S., McKinney, H., Allen, D., & Hall, J. Delivery of community mental health services to black and white clients. *Journal of Consulting and Clinical Psychology,* 1974, *42,* 794–801.

Thomas, A., & Sillen, S. *Racism and psychiatry.* New York: Brunner/Mazel, 1972.

U.S. Department of Commerce, Bureau of the Census. *Current population reports* (Special studies series P-23, No. 80). Washington, D.C.: U.S. Government Printing Office, 1979.

Valentine, C. A. *Culture and poverty: Critique and counterproposals.* Chicago: University of Chicago Press, 1968.

Vontress, C. E. Counseling blacks. *Personnel and Guidance Journal,* 1970, *48,* 713–719.

Wolkon, G. H., Moriwaki, S., & Williams, K. J. Race and social class as factors in the orientation toward psychotherapy. *Journal of Counseling Psychology,* 1973, *20,* 312–316.

Wyatt, G. E., Bass, B. A., & Powell, G. J. A survey of ethnic and sociocultural issues in medical school education. *Journal of Medical Education,* 1978, *53,* 627–632.

Wyatt, G. E., Reardon, D. F., & Bass, B. A. The readjustment of black, high-risk adolescents to the community. *Journal of Community Psychology,* 1977, *5,* 72–78.

Yamamoto, J., James, Q. C., Bloombaum, M., & Hattem, J. Racial factors in patient selection. *American Journal of Psychiatry,* 1967, *124,* 84–90.

CHAPTER 5

On Being Black

Andrea K. Delgado

INTRODUCTION

In psychotherapy, it is often helpful to ask the patient to give an account of a typical day in his or her life. The psychotherapist can gain a more complete view of the patient by examining in detail not only what is stated but also what is left out. For the therapist who may or may not be familiar with the patient's cultural background, such an account will be one way both to develop rapport and also to learn more about the culture from which the patient comes. However, to gain the information, the therapist must know what questions to ask. A simple description of the events will not necessarily provide the answers. The *feelings,* which accompany the events, are of crucial importance.

This chapter will attempt to provide the reader with a view of the daily life experience of blacks, using patient and personal examples. It is hoped that, after reading this chapter, the reader will know even more about the black experience in the United States and how the experience affects the psychotherapeutic process as well as the behavior of blacks.

As noted in Chapter 4, it must be clear that not all blacks are alike. They come from varying socioeconomic, cultural, and familial backgrounds. What is presented here is a composite of the experi-

This chapter does not conform to the self-instructional format of the other chapters because it was felt that its unique style would be compromised. Therefore, read this chapter with the intent to acquire a better perspective of the "feeling" with which black Americans face their daily activities.

ences of men and women of various age groups, various classes, and varying human experiences. Because blacks are people of color, there is a commonality to the black experience that transcends all other variables.

GETTING READY FOR THE DAY

For some people waking up occurs with the help of the radio or television. For one male patient, just beginning the day is the beginning of his daily awareness of being black. The radio tells him about blacks rioting in a major city, enraged at the acquittal of policemen for the alleged beating death of a prominent black executive, and lets him know that the world is not ready for him. And usually the news continues with the latest muggings done by black youths and other crimes. Even though, now, the reporters do not always say the ethnic group from which the perpetrator comes, the image is that it is a black, followed by relief if it turns out not to be. For him, there is an ethnic pride, identity, and embarrassment at 7:40 A.M. each day.

Although the next example comes from a female patient, there is no intent to imply that women are more conscious of their appearance than men. The patient described her daily "ritual" of looking at herself in the mirror and attempting to make her nose less broad, her lips less thick, because that is what she has learned would make her more beautiful. For others, they spend time applying bleaching cream in the morning or at night to lighten their skin. The slogan "Black is beautiful" has aided many a black to develop an image of the beauty of his or her African heritage (Billingsley, 1968). But in the quiet moments in front of the mirror, a black person may still wonder about his or her own attractiveness, and the color of one's skin—how light, how dark—in relation to mother, father, siblings, and other models of beauty.

So the day begins.

GOING TO WORK AND BEING AT WORK

When black persons are at home, they have the shelter of their own environment to protect them from the microaggressions that may confront them once they leave home (Pierce, 1970; Pierce & Allen, 1975). At least with television, radio, and newspaper, they can turn off the switch or throw away the paper even though the memory may have been locked into an internal computer.

A female patient described an example of what appears to be a benign service request. This patient, dressed very neatly, even thinking that that day she looked particularly attractive, stepped outside her apartment to find a taxi to take her to work. Most people have had the experience of waiting endlessly for a taxi. However, what this patient described (with the same rage, frustration, and disappointment she must have felt at the time of the incident) was that empty taxi after taxi passed, some seemingly avoiding her signal, others stopping a half block away to transport a white person. Of course, she finally found a taxi, but her day—her responses to blacks and whites that day—were already predictably tarnished by her experience. The effects on her self-esteem and work performance that day were not measured, but we can assume both were diminished.

Other patients have described the effect of walking into the work place and daily being aware that only a few, or one, black is in a top-level position in the company, or that blacks have the lower- and middle-management positions and there are no blacks at the top. The work environment, viewed as a daily bombardment on blacks, has to leave them with lowered self-esteem, expressed by depression or rage or both but certainly not potentiating their native abilities (Grier & Cobbs, 1968). Such a situation makes it clear that advancement is for the very few, or that there are limits on how far a black person can go, unless he or she is seen as special, serving some "token" function, or superqualified.

The other issue this work scene suggests is the issue of blacks and power. Even if there are a few blacks in top-level positions, power and authority do not always accompany the position: visibility, yes, almost always; power, only sometimes. In categorizing the degree of insult, the taxi incident is a mini-insult, or assault (Pierce, 1970); the absence, or token presence, of blacks with power in the work environment is a maxi-insult to a black person's psyche. But cumulatively, the effect of these daily experiences is devastating.

In every situation in and out of the work setting, a black must factor the effect of race and color into the interaction. Rarely in the United States are there situations where one's blackness is not an issue. An argument with a supervisor, a pay raise, a layoff, a promotion without a pay raise, getting included for lunch, being excluded for lunch, an employee who does not want to be supervised by *you*, the black janitor who only cleans your area out of respect for you and revenge at whites—these are examples of the numerous minute interactions, each requiring some judgment and internal energy and questioning by a black person.

Edwards (1972) describes this process as "minority paranoia." He further describes how minorities "sprout" invisible defensive antennae which pick up clues from a gesture, a tone, a comment and alert the black person to be on guard and suspicious of the other person. He admits that at times this process does not work and mistakes are made but concludes that, in the main, "the occasional misreadings are far less handicapping" than would be the case if blacks gave up their antennae and made themselves vulnerable to the racial trauma which is still inevitable.

STAYING AT HOME

Whether one voluntarily stays at home to take care of children and the house or is out of work or on welfare, for blacks home appears to be a far safer environment than the outside world. For those who work, returning home at the end of the day provides a safe retreat from the outside world. Certainly, in some neighborhoods the possibility of crime and other violence to one's person is a constant threat and makes home not as safe as would otherwise be expected, but it appears that home decreases maxi-insults considerably because by and large personal interactions at home are intraracial rather than interracial.

Television provides both stimulation and pleasure and a source of growing irritation to blacks. Pierce, Carew, Pierce-Gonzalez, and Wills (1977) did a study of television commercials, comparing the number of times blacks and whites are seen and the roles they play in commercials. Pierce *et al.* stated that the average consumer experiences 10,000 commercials each year. By age 12 a child will hear 300,000 commercials, and by grade 12, a child has spent more time before the television than in school. Television can have a powerful impact on molding and maintaining one's identity. The Pierce *et al.* study demonstrated that whites show authority (blacks rarely do); whites dispense favors and goods (blacks have nothing to give); white females are cast as a beauty ideal five times more often than black females, and black males are never so cast. The extent to which racism, sexism, and childism are reflected on television may have decreased somewhat since these data were gathered. However, if it continues to exist in any form, the effect on blacks and whites is to perpetuate attitudes that continue the microaggressions and create a major disability in our society.

JOB-HUNTING

If one ventures to look for a job, again one is faced with the outside world. It is difficult to deal with the feelings of rejection and lowered self-esteem if one does not succeed in obtaining a job right away. There is a double jeopardy for blacks in this situation, sometimes by virtue of lack of opportunity for education and experience and always by virtue of the color of their skin. One female patient, having earnestly spent several months looking for a job, expressed very clearly her ambivalence at continuing to look for one and her willingness to accept her failure to get a job as her own fault. She then asked, "Do you think it's because I'm black?" She was about to use her blackness as a way of not examining her nonracially motivated conflicts, in this case her dependency struggles, and yet it was also likely that she had encountered some racism and sexism in her quest for a position. The latter complicates the therapy and has to be acknowledged, sometimes before the former (internal nonracial conflict) can be addressed.

For a black person the quest for an education can be fraught with many of the same experiences as looking for a job, except that the psychological scars during the child's development and through the educational process may be far greater and have a more far-reaching effect than the adult quest for a job; the former is the antecedent and base of experience for the latter. Pierce (1974) describes this process more fully.

RELATIONSHIPS WITH FAMILY, FRIENDS, AND ACQUAINTANCES

As stated earlier, at-home activities are safer for blacks. It is also true that relationships within the same ethnic group are also safer. One does not have to use the antennae which Edwards describes, for intraracial interactions, both positive and negative, are based on an individual responding to another without the element of racism.

Thus, as is true with other ethnic and cultural groups, there is a tendency to socialize with one's own group. There are shared experiences, jokes, folklore, music, etc. However, in the United States where blacks represent a minority, it is rare that social interactions are solely with one's own group. Today, there are more interracial couples, and there are more interracial social activities than in the past. There are even some subcultures in which there is positive value placed on inviting blacks and other minorities to parties, for example. As might be expected, there can be some suspicion by blacks as to the motivation of such people; however, even with minority paranoia, blacks will venture to such parties and whites to black gatherings (Edwards, 1972).

An observation, yet to be tested, is that blacks whose formative years are spent in a protective, primarily black environment have a greater chance to develop an appropriate dose of self-esteem and positive identity than those who are early confronted with the effects of racism. With mass media, there are likely to be few insulated black communities left. Immigrants from black countries in the Caribbean and in Africa appear to have a healthier sense of self and of their blackness than do those blacks born in the United States.

LEISURE-TIME ACTIVITIES

There is no time, even leisure time, when blacks are not made aware of the effect the color of their skin has on their existence. Even in leisure activities, such as going to the movies, reading magazines, going shopping, and dining out, often the pleasure of the activity is dampened by some microaggression toward them.

For example, such activities may mean waiting in line, having others rush in front of you, witnessing others being served before you and in a different manner (Pierce & Allen, 1975). Reading magazines is similar to watching television: Blacks are rarely visible as an ideal of beauty or occupy roles with less authority than whites or roles that are demeaning, subservient, or attached to myths and stereotypes.

As the black middle class has grown, another form of assault has occurred. At times, whites do not make a distinction between blacks of differing socioeconomic backgrounds. A wealthy young black female patient described an incident in which she went shopping at an expensive boutique. The salesperson took some time before approaching her, and then, when she stated that she liked a particular article of clothing, the salesperson immediately told her the price, as if to discourage her and subtly let her know she could not afford it. This patient said that she could have ruled out the possibility of racial bias, but she was not dressed in a casual manner, and the white patrons were not treated in the same way. Most other immigrants are assimilated into the majority culture over a generation or two, and if they acquire money, the distinctions are few; for a black person, even with money, the shield is not there and the bombardments continue.

CONCLUSION

Not all of the patients' experiences discussed in this chapter will necessarily occur to a single individual in one day. However, the constant bombardment to black persons certainly affects their view of themselves and the world, as well as their attitudes, values, and behavior. Some of the assaults are so minute that over time there is no conscious acknowledgment that they have even occurred. The amount of disease they cause has not been measured. We know about hypertension, increased mortality rates, suicide in black youth, crime, infant mortality rates, poverty, and the loss of black human potential in bettering our society. We do not know all of the effects of negative experiences on black Americans.

Knowledge of the daily, almost unconscious, insults inflicted on blacks by whites, and perpetuated by blacks and whites, will enable the therapist to understand the world of a black person. Values and attitudes do not wait at the door as therapists go into their offices to see a client and resume attachment to the therapist after the session is over.

There are no self-assessment questions and answers based on the content of this chapter. The self-assessment of one's attitudes, values, and behavior is a continuous one. Therapists who are most free of bias, whether black or white, will be able to listen, learn, and treat all their clients appropriately (Gardner, 1972).

REFERENCES

Billingsley, A. *Black families in white America*. Englewood Cliffs, N.J.: Prentice-Hall, 1968.
Edwards, T. J. Looking back on growing up black. In R. Pugh (Ed.), *Psychology and the black experience*. Monterey, Calif.: Brooks/Cole, 1972.
Gardner, L. H. Psychotherapy under varying conditions of race. In R. Pugh (Ed.), *Psychology and the black experience*. Monterey, Calif.: Brooks/Cole, 1972.
Grier, W. H., & Cobbs, P. M. *Black rage*. New York: Basic Books, 1968.
Pierce, C. M. Offensive mechanisms: The vehicle for microaggression. In F. B. Barbour (Ed.), *The black 70's*. Boston: Porter Sargent, 1970.
Pierce, C. M. Psychiatric problems of the black minority. In G. Caplan (Ed.), *American handbook of psychiatry*. New York: Basic Books, 1974.
Pierce, C. M., & Allen, G. B. Childism. *Psychiatric Annals*, 1975, 5, 15–24.
Pierce, C. M., Carew, J. V., Pierce-Gonzalez, D., & Wills, D. An experiment in racism: TV commercials. *Education and Urban Society*, 1977, 10, 61–87.

CHAPTER 6

Asian-American and Pacific-Islander Patients

Ching-piao Chien and Joe Yamamoto

INTRODUCTION

The issue of mental health for Asian Americans and Pacific Islanders has been relatively neglected over the last decades for several reasons. First, they are the minority of minorities. Second, Orientals, particularly the Chinese in Chinatown, are stereotyped as tranquil and well disciplined; the low incidence of juvenile delinquency, crime, alcoholism, and divorce in Chinatown has often misled the public into believing that there is no serious mental health problem among this population (Sue, 1977). Third, the common notion of the "inscrutable Oriental" makes Asian Americans less attractive to the mental health professional than the YAVIS (young, attractive, verbal, intelligent, and successful) patients (Schofield, 1964). Fourth, there are relatively few bilingual and bicultural mental health professionals to present the unique problems of Asian Americans to the remaining majority of professionals. Fifth, until the middle of the 20th century, there has been no political representation for Asian Americans and Pacific Islanders at the congressional, or cabinet level by Asian Americans or Pacific Islanders. Finally, it is only in the last few years that mandatory priority has been given to the minorities through legislation, executive order, or court opinion. President Reagan's budget reductions have had a heavy impact on these improvements and we fear that the net result will be the loss of all these gains for the minorities.

In 1978, the Presidential Commission on Mental Health clearly pointed out that mental health and services for minorities should be considered a priority. Special training funds have been made available through the National Institute of Mental Health for psychiatric residency and psychology training facilities willing to provide such programs for these priority patients. Other priority patients include the elderly, children, and chronic mental patients.

In the Asian-American and Pacific-Islander populations, these categories also need particular attention. Fortunately, American psychiatry, psychology, and mental health groups have just begun to address serious deficiencies in the care of these groups, regardless of ethnic background. Close collaboration with all researchers and service providers engaging in the care of the various ethnic groups of the priority categories should be promoted simultaneously in order to maximize efficiency.

The information in this chapter is based on both published data and unpublished observation of the special problems of Asian-American and Pacific-Islander patients. It should be noted that many of the descriptions of the Asian American character traits contained in this chapter are both quantitative and qualitative. Mental health issues affecting Asian Americans and Pacific Islanders have long been neglected; consequently the research and clinical data are extremely deficient. The authors hope that this chapter will stimulate further thought and studies in the mental health delivery system for Asian Americans and Pacific Islanders.

By the time readers have completed this chapter and a corresponding group discussion session, we expect readers to be able to:

1. Describe the sociocultural characteristics of Asian Americans which may affect the service they receive at a psychiatric outpatient clinic or mental health facility
2. Describe the important attitudes of Asian Americans toward mental health services
3. Discuss the most common problems faced by therapists when treating Asian Americans
4. Describe and use therapeutic approaches which are most effective with Asian-American patients
5. Express satisfaction with the process and outcome of therapeutic encounters with Asian-American patients

Please read the above learning objectives until you become familiar with the goals of this chapter; then continue reading.

CHARACTERISTICS OF ASIAN AMERICANS AND PACIFIC ISLANDERS

Demographic Characteristics

Although there are some striking similarities among all minority and low-income groups, Asian Americans and Pacific Islanders exhibit unique diversities and complexities in their respective demographic characteristics. Asian Americans and Pacific Islanders of more than 20 different ethnic backgrounds are now residing in the United States, each with different languages, religions, and socioeconomic levels. They represent a microcosm of the vast Asian Pacific region in which more than one-quarter of the entire world population live, including some of the world's most affluent and most deprived nations. Immigrants from these sociocultural and geographical backgrounds would certainly create significant heterogeneous groups even though they are termed singularly as Asian Americans and Pacific Islanders.

The complexities are compounded when one considers different generations and degrees of acculturation. For the most part, the new immigrants think and behave in their native manner, almost identically to the people in their home country. The second generation often receive their education in the American school system, speak English in the vernacular, and yet still maintain their cultural heritage, which is received at home from immigrant parents. Later generations are much closer to Anglo-Americans in their English proficiency and value systems. At this point, even though they are of similar racial background, they are often no longer bilingual and are certainly a very different entity from their first-generation ethnic counterparts.

It is the less acculturated groups that need particular attention, consideration, and culturally sensitive services when their problems arise. They are often caught in a state of helplessness, without appropriate social support systems. Resources that they would have relied on in their home countries are often not found in the United States, while the existing resources may appear alien to them. In addition to various adaptational problems faced by legal immigrants, illegal aliens encounter a number of obvious social, psychological, and legal problems.

Not uncommonly, many aliens of Asian or Pacific-Island background view their status in the United States as merely a station in their life's journey. Many of them choose to come to the United States for political, educational, and financial advantages but often hope one day to return to their home country. Some aliens still maintain citizenship in their home country and never become naturalized, although they have lived in the United States for several decades. Even among those who were naturalized or are second-generation, some still plan to return to their roots—to their "home country." Such a view often perpetuates their alien status and hinders integration into American society. These people tend to live in their ethnic ghettos, stick resolutely to their ethnic life-styles, continue to speak in their native language, and barely speak English. They often do not vote and are apathetic to political movements. This could be reflected by their attitude in calling fellow Americans "those Americans" with a tone implying national boundaries within the United States. On the other hand, there are some Asians who seek naturalization as quickly as possible, Americanize their names, do not live in ghettos, intermarry with whites, and identify themselves more closely with the majority Americans. Between these two groups is the third group, which claims equal rights and privileges with American citizens yet retains its cultural heritage with pride. People in this group often call themselves Chinese American, Japanese American, Korean American, and so forth, including both their Asian and American heritage (Sue & Sue, 1974). Therefore, an individual's identification indeed would create a different psychosocial status of Asian Americans even though they are the same generation and of the same ethnic group.

The recent influx of Indochinese refugees creates another factor for the complexity of Asian-American immigration. According to U.S. State Department estimates of refugees in the year 1980, there are 168,000 Indochinese mostly from Vietnam and Cambodia. They rank number one among the four major refugee categories in 1980, the others being Cuba (117,000); Soviet Union and East Europe (50,000); and Haiti (15,000) (Adler, Lord, Newhall, McGuire, & Coppola, 1980). The United States is unprepared both culturally and socially for this sudden influx, as are the refugees.

There have been feelings of hostility and rivalry by other minorities toward this new group in terms of job competition and sharing of financial support from federal resources. Those Americans who are burdened with high taxes and spiralling welfare costs have expressed their resentment at feeding these refugees while there are other pressing matters unattended. Although eventually these traumatized refugees will be granted citizenship, their psychosocial experiences as new Asian Americans will certainly be different from those who are acculturated and well integrated in American suburbs.

Languages

Most Asian Americans are of Chinese, Japanese, Korean, Filipino, Vietnamese, Cambodian, Laotian, or Samoan origin, each with their different languages. Although Japanese, Korean, and Vietnamese involve certain Chinese characters, pronunciation has been altered and thus assimilated into their native language. Even within one ethnic group, such as the Chinese, there are several dialects: Cantonese is significantly different from Fukienese, which is spoken by the majority of Taiwanese; Cantonese can be further subdivided into several village dialects. In the Japanese language there is a notable difference in accent and expression between eastern (*kanto*) and western (*kansai*) people. However, because of recent efforts in compulsory education using the national standard language, serious language barriers within each Asian country have been much alleviated. Non–English-speaking Asian Americans still cannot communicate from one group to the other. However, among the native-born Chinese, Japanese, Korean and older Vietnamese, Chinese characters—though pronounced differently—may provide a means for communication.

Religion and Philosophy

Buddhism is the most popular religion among Chinese, Koreans, Indochinese, and Japanese. Shintoism is the national religion of the Japanese, while Taoism is quite prevalent among Chinese, Koreans, and Indochinese (ethnic Chinese). The Philippines has been significantly influenced by Catholicism because of the Spanish colonization. Because of the relative scarcity of Buddhist and Taoist temples and Shinto shrines in the United States, these religious activities are mostly carried out on a limited scale. Christianity, on the other hand, appears to grow readily in the European-American cultural soil. In Los Angeles, for instance, there are more than 200 Christian churches in the Korean community actively affecting community affairs. Native

Koreans are 40% Christian. Among the recently immigrated Taiwanese, regular church gatherings have become one of the most viable communication networks. The role of the clergy is therefore, understandably important in planning and delivering community mental health services. Appropriate involvement of such a network could provide valuable human resources for mental health programs.

Confucianism, often misunderstood as a religion, is an important philosophical discipline which has deeply affected the majority of Asians. It is a doctrine taught by one of the world's greatest philosophers and teachers, Confucius (Kung-tzu), about 500 years before the birth of Christ. Confucianism basically consists of five fundamental ethics: (1) loyalty between the lord and his subordinates (in this modern era, this can be interpreted as loyalty betweeen the employer and employee); (2) intimacy between father and son; (3) propriety between husband and wife; (4) order between elder and junior; and (5) trust between friends. These five ethics are deeply rooted in the everyday life of the Chinese, Japanese, Koreans, and Vietnamese. Even Filipinos are considerably affected by Confucianism because of the Chinese who immigrated to the Philippines. These ethics have become the backbone of human relationships. Confucian emphasis on filial piety contributed to the formation of Asian characteristics such as respect for parents and seniors, obedience, and close family ties. These personality traits are considered desirable virtues in the Confucian-dominated culture, yet often appear to be "passive-aggressive," "nonassertive," or "overly submissive to authority" in the eye of those who are not familiar with Confucianism. A culturally sensitive insight is important because it is relevant to the conduct of family therapy, to the interpretation of psychotherapeutic content and process, and to understanding Asian family life.

Now complete the Self-Assessment Exercise 6.1.

SELF-ASSESSMENT EXERCISE 6.1

1. List at least four characteristics of Asian Americans who are currently living in the United States but who plan eventually to return to their homeland.

    a.
    b.
    c.
    d.

2. List at least three characteristics of Asian Americans who are currently living in the United States and intend to stay.

    a.
    b.
    c.
    d.

3. List the four major religions practiced by Asian Americans.

    a.
    b.
    c.
    d.

4. Asian Americans who follow the Confucian philosophy may be diagnosed as _____ or _____ by American therapists because _____

When you have completed this exercise, check your answers with those that follow.

SELF-ASSESSMENT EXERCISE 6.1: FEEDBACK

1. Asian Americans planning to return to their home country:

   a. maintain citizenship in the home country
   b. live in ethnic ghettos
   c. maintain the ethnic life-style
   d. speak their native language but no English
   e. do not vote and are apathetic to political movements
   f. remain isolated from mainstream American life

2. Asian Americans planning to stay:

   a. Americanize their ethnic name
   b. live in nonethnic neighborhoods
   c. intermarry with European Americans
   d. identify with the majority Americans

3. The major religions are:
   a. Buddhism
   b. Shintoism
   c. Taoism
   d. Catholicism

4. Asian Americans who follow the Confucian philosophy may be diagnosed as "passive-aggressive," "nonassertive," or "overly submissive to authority" by American therapists because Confucianism has contributed greatly to the Asians' deep respect for parents and seniors, obedient behavior, and close family ties.

If your answers correspond closely with those above, continue your reading. Otherwise, reread the preceding material.

ATTITUDES TOWARD MENTAL HEALTH SERVICES

It is interesting to note that in attitudes toward mental health services there are striking similarities between Asian Americans, poor and working-class patients, and Hispanic Americans. Although the general attitudes of ethnic minorities toward mental health services might appear to be the same, there are certain cultural roots among Asian Americans that cause unique problems.

Influence of Confucianism

It is well known that the Confucian doctrine, "While there are no stirrings of pleasure, anger, sorrow and joy, the mind may be said to be in the state of tranquility" (Legge, 1973), has influenced remarkably the affective expression of Asians in the past centuries. To most of the European Americans, not surprisingly, Asians with reduced affective tone appear to be "inscrutable." One can understand readily that it is not within the cultural norm for Asians to reveal and discuss their emotions in public and to strangers although Koreans may be the exception to this rule (Yamamoto & Steinberg, 1981). Mental health services are often viewed by Asians as facilities for "crazy people" who are "psychotic" and cannot control their own lives. To discuss problems-of-life situations—marriage, job, school, friends, family, and especially sex—with the mental health worker is quite ego-alien to most Asians. If forced to behave like the majority of Americans, they will see this as a realistic threat and often terminate the therapy prematurely. Such culture-bound attitudes, coupled with the commonly held stigma attached to mental illness, have led to the underutilization of mental health services not only in their native countries but also in the United States. Underutilization has occurred here despite tremendous efforts to promote a mental health movement by two American presidents, with vast amounts of federal, state, county, and private funds being poured into mental health services (Kinsey, 1974; Mochizuki, 1975; Sue & McKinney, 1975).

Biological, Spiritual, and Moralistic Views

Some Asians and Pacific Islanders still believe that mental illness stems from either "bad blood" or "evil" as the Europeans did in past centuries. Buddhists or Taoists would interpret mental illness as a manifestation of a "sin" that the patient's ancestor committed generations ago. Whether mental illness is attributed to biological, spiritual, or moralistic causes, it all will result in "losing face" and ostracism. Patients' relatives often encounter very serious obstacles in dating, marriage, social life, and employment in their own community. The price a family has to pay for having a mental patient is so high that it is understandable that the family would try to keep problems secret and within the family circle. This often leads to a delay in case detection and early therapeutic intervention. Commonly, Asians appear in the clinic either in an emergency state (life or death situation) or in a full-blown psychotic state which is beyond the family's control (Fung, Uchalik, Lo, Reece, & Lam, 1980). Concealing the mental illness within the family circle is not all negative. Appropriate usage of such an attitude may facilitate effective home treatment and family therapy. Home treatment needs to be encouraged.

Need for Innovative Approaches

Using innovative and practical ways to approach the emotionally distressed, reluctant Asian population should be one of the top priorities in the planning of mental health delivery systems. Some basic information on the prevalence of mental illness among Asian Americans and Pacific Islanders is essential to achieve such a goal. Extensive epidemiological studies on the prevalence, incidence, outcome, and causative factors of mental illness among these complex and diversified populations would provide theoretical and rational grounds for future planning. Unfortunately, such information is seriously lacking at the present. Although the total number of Asian Americans and Pacific Islanders is relatively smaller than that of other minorities and, therefore, logistically easier for an epidemiological survey, the ever-changing population, resulting from recent changes in the political and socioeconomic status of the Pacific Asian, has caused difficulties in methodology and the updating of findings.

PROBLEMS IN TREATING ASIAN-AMERICAN AND PACIFIC-ISLANDER PATIENTS

Unfamiliarity with Appointment System

Most new immigrants have been accustomed to first-come, first-served walk-in clinics in their native countries. Such a system has been widely practiced in private and public clinical facilities for generations. In Japan, Taiwan, and Southeast Asia, it is not uncommon for a practicing physician to see more than 100 patients a day on a walk-in basis. This is a striking contrast to the U.S. mental health facilities, in which only a few patients can be seen in a day because of the appointment system.

Although scheduled visits will assure enough time for the patients and therapists as well, it is often a shock for less acculturated Asians to find out that the visit to the therapist is not totally under their own control, but more or less dependent on the available time of the therapist. As mentioned before, Asians use health facilities on an emergency basis and not so much for prevention. If the appointment system causes delayed contact with the therapist, this creates frustration and disappointment. They may not show up for the appointment if the earlier crisis and tension have subsided during the waiting period. Thorough explanations on the positive aspects of the appointment system to the patient and the therapist's willingness to maintain flexibility for the patient's visiting time could quickly gain the patient's rapport in the initial contacts.

History Taking

Detailed history taking is a mandate in U.S. clinical facilities as stipulated by the Joint Commission on the Accreditation of Hospitals. Particularly in psychiatry, history taking in the initial interview includes chief complaints, present illness, past history, developmental history covering early childhood experiences, psychosexual, vocational, social, financial, familial, and marital histories, and so forth. Heavy emphasis is placed on the assessment of the patient's biological, psychological, social, educational, vocational, recreational, and cultural needs. Such history taking is both time-consuming and painstaking for patients and health workers.

If the Asian patient is non–English-speaking, the experience will be extremely frustrating for the mental health clinician and client alike. Even if the clinician speaks the client's native language, such an intensive interview in the initial contact nonetheless often creates a negative therapeutic relationship.

Asians and Pacific Islanders who have sought help from folk healers in the past are accustomed to their intuitive, nonverbal approaches. For instance, Chinese herb doctors make their diagnoses by touching the pulse, feeling the warmth of the skin, looking at the eyes of the patient—all within about two minutes. They then start prescribing herbs without the intensive history taking practiced by American clinicians. As a matter of fact, there is a common belief among Chinese patients that the fewer questions herb doctors and folk healers ask about patients' problems, the more capable and perceptive they are. Just by touching, feeling, and looking at the patient, competent herb doctors and folk healers are expected to diagnose the problems of the present and even of the past.

Young children may be reminded by their mother not to speak a word when they are examined by an herb doctor. If the herb medicine the doctor prescribes happens to be effective in managing the illness within a few days, the herb doctor will then be highly praised for being able to read everything from his pulse-touching diagnostic technique.

Therefore, the lengthy questions the clinician asks about past and present history may make it appear to the patient that the clinician is incompetent. The following anecdotal episode of the transaction between an Asian patient and an American clinician is a true story.

CLINICIAN: What is your problem?
PATIENT: If I knew my problem, I wouldn't have come here.

As mentioned before, most Asian Americans and Pacific Islanders visit clinics mostly on an emergency basis. They expect the therapist to relieve their pain and agony with action, not with extensive history taking. If the clinician is insensitive to these patients' orientations and expectations and tries to enforce a routine procedure of the clinic on them, it will probably create distrust and loss of faith on the patients' part. It is advisable, therefore, that the therapist focus more on the symptom relief and problem management during the first few sessions. Once the patient is convinced that the clinician can serve his or her immediate needs, then thorough history taking can follow without much resistance.

Laboratory Tests

Because of malpractice suits, American doctors often overprescribe laboratory tests. To many less educated Asian Americans and Pacific Islanders, blood appears to be the very essence of life. A routine lab test may appear to be overtaxing to the patient. Two or three test tubes of blood, which are routinely drawn in the American clinical laboratory for the complete blood count, biochemical profile, and liver function test, may be perceived as a threat to vitality by some patients. Even psychological testing and extensive interviewing for the computer analysis of psychopathology would be seen by patients as procedures irrelevant to their immediate needs. Again, without careful explanation of the purpose of such a procedure and appropriate timing to carry out these tests, clinicians may often lose their patients without knowing why.

Medical Model

The roles of the clinical psychologist, psychiatric social worker, and nurse in Asian countries are quite different from those found in the American scene. In the United States, professionals from these different disciplines take active roles in the diagnostic interview, treatment, planning, and psychotherapeutic treatment. The less acculturated Asian Americans are not accustomed to being treated solely by professionals from these disciplines without seeing a physician. Several reports have pointed out that many psychiatric problems of Asians and Pacific Islanders are manifested with somatic complaints, particularly in the case of depression. Even the symptom of anxiety, which is primarily psychological, is often attributed by these patients to a defect in the kidney, hormonal imbalance, or malnutrition. Some Chinese believe this is due to excessive *yang* in the liver (meaning too much fire in the liver). Therefore, their expectation of treatment is often a medical solution with a medicinal and physical approach.

Psychotherapy or talk therapy hardly exists in their native culture as it has in the United States. For instance, what we call group psychotherapy in the United States is described as "mass education" in China and "group dialogue" only recently in Japan.

A Harvard-trained Taiwanese psychiatrist returned to practice psychotherapy in Taiwan several years ago. He encountered serious resistance from his patients in collecting fees because the patients felt they hadn't received treatment other than "talking." This example clearly illustrates the need for thorough explanation of the nature and purpose of psychotherapy. Only when patients understand talking therapy as a treatment modality can the therapist initiate a psychotherapeutic contract.

Now complete the Self-Assessment Exercise 6.2.

SELF-ASSESSMENT EXERCISE 6.2

Describe as completely as you can typical Asian-American attitudes and reactions to the following areas.

1. Mental illness

2. The appointment system

3. The history-taking procedures

4. Laboratory tests

5. Talking psychotherapy

When you have completed this exercise, check your answers with those that follow.

1. Mental illness
   For many Asian Americans, mental illness is regarded as a result of bad blood or sin and will result in "losing face" and ostracism. Mental patients and family members encounter very serious obstacles in dating, marriage, social life, and employment. The social and personal price is so high that problems are usually kept at home until they are out of hand.

2. The appointment system
   Asians are more accustomed to report for treatment when they are feeling bad and expect a first-come, first-served system. The American system of appointments tends to delay the immediacy of treatment, and they generally do not like it.

3. The history-taking procedures
   Asian Americans are not likely to discuss problems in marriage, job, school, friends, family, or sex with a mental health worker. They are sometimes more accustomed to folk healers who simply touch, feel, and look at patients and then prescribe treatment. Typically, patients do not describe why they are there. Questions make the Asian patient feel the therapist is incompetent, and therefore too many early questions may cause the patient to withdraw from therapy.

4. Laboratory tests
   Laboratory tests for urine and blood are looked at with suspicion; they may appear to be irrelevant.

5. Talking psychotherapy
   Most Asian Americans are accustomed to being treated in a physical way or advised in a parental way. In general they must be gradually led to accept talking therapies.

If your answers correspond closely with those above, continue reading. Otherwise, reread the preceding material.

SPECIAL CONSIDERATIONS IN THERAPEUTIC APPROACHES

Psychotherapy

Psychotherapy in the United States began with the contributions of Sigmund Freud, Alfred Adler, Carl Jung, and Adolf Meyer. All were Europeans dealing basically with middle-class European patient populations, beginning from the time of Queen Victoria's reign in Great Britain. Thus, the problems presented were those of conflicts related to rigid Victorian values.

The values of patients of Asian background have many similarities to Victorian values because of the more rigid, hierarchical, and structured nature of their societies. As a matter of fact, many characteristics of Asian Americans and Pacific Islanders in the 1980s could be found in European Americans around the turn of the century. Despite these similarities, there are now differences with modern-day white Americans. Table 6.1 compares the characteristics of Asian and white Americans.

Quantitative and qualitative differences should be kept in mind when the therapist is going to initiate psychotherapy with Asian

Table 6.1. Comparison of Asian-American and White American Attitudes and Values

Attitude/value	Asian Americans	White Americans
Family ties	Very strong	Relatively loose
Extended family	Common	Uncommon; mostly nuclear family
Respect for authority	Great	Less
Respect for tradition	Great	Less
Concern about the relationship with others	Great emphasis on the relationships with parents, spouses, siblings, and extended kinship	Emphasis on individualism, self-development, self-achievement, and self-growth
Adherence to the medical model	Often expect the physician to treat with medicinal agents; emotional problems presented in somatic symptoms	Often reluctant to take psychotropic medication; more readily accept psychotherapy or counseling from nonmedical clinician
Company of family members in clinic visits	Often; confidentiality is not so important among family members	Less; confidentiality and private talk is important even in the same family
Expectation on the goal of treatment	Symptomatic relief, short treatment course	Change of coping, long-term treatment
Therapist's role	Authority figure	Neutral, nonjudgmental, noncritical, blank screen
Openness to emotional problems	Closed	Open

patients. Strong family ties, respect for authority and tradition, great emphasis on family relationships, different attitudes toward emotional problems and psychiatric treatment, and so on, call for special consideration in planning psychotherapy.

The Family versus the Individual. In most Asian and Pacific cultures, the family is the important unit, not the individual. This emphasis on the family and social relationships contrasts starkly with the extreme emphasis on the individual and independence in the United States. This has consequences for the psychotherapeutic approach: a family-oriented psychotherapy may be much more appropriate for nonacculturated Asians and Pacific Islanders. Third- and fourth-generation Asian Americans and Pacific Islanders usually insist on an individual and independent psychotherapeutic approach, just like other Americans.

The Role of the Psychotherapist. In the United States, the psychotherapist is expected to be democratic and equal to the patient. Conceptually, this is important because Americans live in a democratic society and are socialized to exercise their roles as citizens on an equal basis. In contrast, most Asians and Pacific Islanders come from societies where there is a vertical structure. Thus, an Asian or Pacific patient who is not acculturated to American democratic values might feel insecure and anxious if the therapist were to behave in a democratic and egalitarian manner. For this reason, the therapist must adopt a much more authoritative attitude, assuming an air of self-confidence and understanding of the patient's problems. Like a good parent, the therapist must behave in an authoritative manner, with a clear understanding of the therapist's role. In assuming the authority, the therapist should remember that the patient's family is a resource and can form part of a therapeutic team working to improve the defined patient's health.

Therapist Activity versus Therapist Passivity. In American psychotherapy, there has been considerable emphasis on the therapist as a neutral, nonjudgmental, noncritical, relatively passive person. In contrast, Asians and Pacific Islanders need therapists to assume the role of authority figure in order to actively engage in the therapeutic process. Thus, it would not be appropriate to wait endlessly for the patient to unravel his or her history and to define the problems. As mentioned before, some patients are used to traditional Chinese practitioners who are expected merely to check the pulse of the patient and then diagnose and treat the patient's illness. The expectations of the Asian patient will be high in terms of the therapist's immediate understanding and knowledge of the patient's problems. Although we may resist such instant insight and understanding, it is important to convey an air of confidence and understanding.

Active Empathy versus Neutral Mirror. Among Asian and Pacific patients, there is a yearning for an actively empathic parental figure (Yamamoto, 1980). This conflicts very strongly with the concept of the neutral mirrorlike therapist who merely reflects what the patient is saying. This is a very prevalent cultural expectation. Professor Takeo Doi, who trained at the Menninger Foundation, tells a story about how he was invited to a friend's home in Topeka, Kansas. The friend asked Professor Doi, "Are you hungry? Would you like something to eat?" Doi responded, "No, thank you." He assumed that the host would do as a Japanese host would, that is, assume that he was hungry, offer him something specific to eat rather than the open-ended question which would have been unacceptable in Japan. Here an empathic host would have said, "You must be hungry, here is some ice cream," or "I'm sure that you have room to enjoy a little bit of dessert." Although American psychotherapists very much emphasize the importance of empathy, we have chosen the phrase "active empathy" to point out that not only must psychotherapists try to put themselves in their patients' shoes and really understand what their patients feel and what the problems are, but also they must then try to do something that will be helpful in relieving the symptoms or the problems.

Brief versus Long-Term Considerations. Asian patients frequently have the medical model in mind. Because of this, they hope to have the problem or symptoms relieved by visiting the doctor. The usual conceptualization of treatment is short term. Thus, the medical model with the emphasis on symptomatic relief fits the situation much better for Asian Americans and Pacific Islanders with their brief time orientation and focus on the improvement of symptoms or the problems. This contrasts significantly with the picture that American psychotherapists have of the importance of insight or self-understanding as the objective of psychotherapy.

Other Considerations. In considering Asian Americans and Pacific Islanders, it is important to be aware of their heterogeneity and ethnic differences. For example, Koreans are much more outgoing than Japanese. In addition, one must consider the generation of the patient, for an unacculturated Chinese-American patient may be quite different than a third- or fourth-generation Chinese American. Social class needs to be taken into account. Many of the original immigrants from Asia tended to come from the farming classes. As such, they had the limited education of most farmers and so would be unsophisticated about mental health. More recently, immigrants from South Korea, Taiwan, and the Philippines have been upper-middle-class professionals. Their knowledge of and sophistication about mental health services is superior to that of the average white American in the United States. We have seen first-generation Filipinos who came for therapy who behaved like white Americans.

Geographic location is another important factor. In the state of Hawaii, Asian Americans comprise the majority. Government officials are mostly Asian Americans, and they are well represented in the middle classes. The officials and dignitaries are good role models. In contrast, social support in Midwestern communities for most Asian-American and Pacific-Islander populations may be difficult to obtain. Chicago and New York, of course, have substantial Asian-American populations.

Thus, the appropriate therapy for a particular patient varies from thoroughly modified treatment appropriate for unacculturated Asian Americans to the routine sort of therapy offered to most majority Americans. Acculturated Asian-American populations would be included in the latter group; for them verbal expressiveness is increased and acceptance of psychotherapy is greater.

Now complete the Self-Assessment Exercise 6.3.

SELF-ASSESSMENT EXERCISE 6.3

Describe the attitudes which best reflect the attitudes and values of the Asian American and the white American.

Attitude/value	Asian American	White American
Family ties		
Concern about the relationship with others		
Adherence to the medical model		
Company of family members in clinic visits		
Expectation on the goal of treatment		
Therapist's role		
Openness to emotional problems		

When you have completed this exercise, check your answers with those that follow.

SELF-ASSESSMENT EXERCISE 6.3: FEEDBACK

The attitudes which best reflect the attitudes and values of the Asian American and the white American include:

Attitude/value	Asian American	White American
Family ties	Very strong	Relatively loose
Concern about the relationship with others	Great emphasis on the relationships with parents, spouses, siblings, and extended kinships	Emphasis on individualism, self-development, self-achievement, and self-growth
Adherence to the medical model	Often expect the physician to treat with medicinal agents; emotional problems presented in somatic symptoms	Often reluctant to take psychotropic medication; more readily accept psychotherapy or counseling from nonmedical clinician
Company of family members in clinic visits	Often; confidentiality is not so important among family members	Less; confidentiality and private talk is important even in the same family
Expectation on the goal of treatment	Symptomatic relief, short treatment course	Change of coping, long-term treatment
Therapist's role	Active authority figure	Neutral, nonjudgmental, noncritical, blank screen
Openness to emotional problems	Closed	Open

If your answers correspond closely with those above, continue reading. Otherwise, reread the preceding material.

Pharmacotherapy

For most Asian Americans who are medically and somatically oriented, medicinal treatment implies special healing power. The role

138

and appropriate utilization of pharmacotherapy, therefore, is particularly important in the psychiatric treatment of Asian Americans. Unfortunately, almost all of the psychotropic drugs now available in the United States were made in Western countries, and the test subjects were from non-Asian populations. The data, such as dosage range, safety, and side effects, are mostly based on European or American populations. Clinical reports from Asian countries, and sporadic reports in the United States regarding the drug response of Asian patients, suggest that the data based on Caucasian populations may not be readily applicable to the Asian population. Common reports indicate that Asian patients require a lower dosage, manifest side effects readily with low or medium "American dosage," and show sensitivity to drugs with anticholinergic properties (such as tricyclic antidepressants and neuroleptics). Although the question of whether or not cultural adaptation with change in diet and climate affects the drug response still remains to be answered, some data from Asian countries suggest that Asians do require smaller doses of medication.

Dosage. In general, the maximum dosage of neuroleptics for Asian patients does not exceed 500 mg of chlorpromazine and its dosage equivalence for other neuroleptics. The initial dosage can be 50 to 100 mg b.i.d. for acute psychotic patients. Some patients sleep more than 12 hours just from 50 mg chlorpromazine intramuscularly. Postural hypotension, oculogyric crisis, and other types of dystonia are commonly observed in the first few days of medication even at low dosage.

Yamashita and Asano (1979) surveyed 10 Asian countries by questionnaire and found relatively low dosages of antidepressants used in the treatment of endogenous depression, a finding similar to the experience of Yamamoto, Fung, Lo, and Reece (1979) in the Los Angeles Asian/Pacific Counseling and Treatment Center. The average range of imipramine in Asia is 70–134 mg or 1.4–2.7 mg/kgm, as compared to 3.5 mg/kgm in Glassman and Roose's (1979) study involving white patients in New York. The dosage ratio between Asian and white patients is thus roughly 1:2 when the common clinical practice of using 250–300 mg or higher daily dosage of imipramine in the United States is considered. The plasma levels of Japanese patients are proportionate to their oral dosage, that is, smaller dosages yield lower plasma levels. In 17 of 21 Japanese patients with successful therapeutic outcome, the plasma level (imipramine and desipramine combined) was below 100 ng/ml as compared to 180 ng/ml and above in Glassman and Roose's Occidental population. A similar trend was found in amitriptyline-treated patients—20 of 26 patients showed the plasma level of amitriptyline and nortriptyline combined to be 65 ng/ml and below.

Takahashi's (1978) review of the lithium treatment of affective disorders in Japan again revealed a similar pattern as is the case with tricyclic antidepressants. Nearly 70% of Japanese manic patients responded to lithium with a plasma level below 0.86 mEq/liter, while 0% responded at such a level in a United States collaborative study. As to depression, Japanese patients responded at 0.41 mEq/liter, while United States patients required a plasma level higher than 0.7 mEq/liter.

Honda and Suzuki's (1979) study of saliva lithium in Japan discloses a highly significant correlation between saliva and plasma lithium concentration (saliva–plasma ratio = 2.62 ± 0.84), a finding close to that in the United States (2.26 ± 0.23); in Germany (2.13 ± 0.31); and in India (2.22 ± 0.50). This may suggest that the basic physiological mechanisms of excreting lithium are quite universal, regardless of race or culture. However, Honda and Suzuki's comment that relatively higher values of volume of distribution (Vd) and renal clearance (Cl Li) are found in the United States than those in Japan needs further clarification.

Lastly, in their review of 31 papers, Georgotas and Gershon (1979) came to the conclusion that:

> Relationship between plasma lithium level and effective maintenance treatment has not been well explored and none of the reported long-term studies have provided a definite answer regarding this issue. All studies except one utilize plasma levels but none was a plasma level-response study with patients randomly assigned to various plasma levels. Their recommended levels for effective maintenance treatment are quite variable and are mainly based on post hoc analysis of data . (p. 37)

In view of the possible renal interstitial fibrosis associated with long-term usage of lithium, minimum optimal dosage should be established with the plasma level as an indicator.

In conclusion, more data are now available than ever before with standard laboratory measurements of psychopathology and of plasma levels of lithium and tricyclic antidepressants. The current therapeutic plasma level of lithium, as well as of tricyclic antidepressants used in the United States, does not appear to be applicable to the Japanese population. Whether this is due to receptor sensitivity or to a socio-cultural factor, such as difference in tolerance to psychopathology, needs to be further investigated. Rational, safe, and economic treatment regimens can only be established once such answers are available (Chien, 1979).

Side Effects. The common side effect of all psychotropic drugs—neuroleptics, antidepressants, lithium, and even antianxiety agents—is akinesia, a syndrome characterized by weakness of the muscles and extremities. This side effect, if not appropriately explained beforehand, could be easily misinterpreted by Asian patients as deficiency in their vital strength. They may either refuse to continue the medication or seek some herbs, tonics, vitamins, or even hormones to improve their "vitality." The latter substances are often self-administered and are not known to the treating physician or therapist. Possible interactions between these self-medications and prescribed psychotropic drugs could sometimes be dangerous to the patient's health, if not fatal, and could sometimes be mind-altering. Such a secret self-medication may obscure the treatment course and puzzle the therapist as to the cause of paradoxical outcome. Educational effort should be made to stop such a practice by the patient or family members.

Frequency of Medication. Some patients with limited education may believe the more often they take medication, the faster they improve. Therefore, they overmedicate themselves. On the other hand, if physicians prescribe three or four times a day, some working patients or less concerned patients may forget one or two of their regular medication times, the end result being undermedication. The latter case is really unnecessary because most psychotropic drugs have quite long half-lives and can reasonably be administered once or twice a day. Careful thought about the medication schedule best tailored to meet the individual's life-style, working schedule, and pharmacological rationale is important.

Economic Considerations. The therapist should be concerned about the financial burden which medications may impose on patients, particularly on the poor. There are many drugs that are not covered by Medicare or Medicaid. The cost of the drug could be a special burden, since medication often requires a lengthy treatment. The prescribing physician may help the patient to cut the cost of drugs by choosing large dosage tablets instead of smaller dosage tablets. For example, if the patient is taking 400 mg/day of thioridazine, it can be administered in several ways, such as four 25 mg tablets q.i.d., or one 200 mg tablet b.i.d. Since the cost of the larger dosage tablet is only slightly higher than the smaller dosage tablet, the savings could be substantial if the prescription is made with one 200 mg. tablet b.i.d. instead of four 25 mg. tablets q.i.d. Further, since the patents of several popular psychotropic drugs have now expired, equally effective generic drugs are now being marketed at a substantially lower cost.

Now complete the Self-Assessment Exercise 6.4.

SELF-ASSESSMENT EXERCISE 6.4

1. Why is it so important to explain to Asian patients the potential side effects of psychotropic drugs?

2. Give two reasons why it may be advisable to prescribe medication dosages which require the patient to take medication just once or twice a day.

   a.

   b.

When you have completed this exercise, check your answers with those that follow.

SELF-ASSESSMENT EXERCISE 6.4: FEEDBACK

1. It is important to explain to Asian patients the potential side effects of psychotropic drugs because Asian patients may interpret the possible weakness in muscles and extremities as a deficiency in their vital strength and therefore may self-administer herbs, tonics, or other substances, and this will lead to paradoxical outcomes.

2. It may be advisable to prescribe medication dosages which require the patient to take medication just once or twice a day because:

   a. Taking medication once or twice a day is easier to remember than taking medication three or four times a day

   b. One large tablet costs less than several small tablets which, when combined, equal the dosage of the larger tablet

If your answers correspond closely with those above, continue your reading. Otherwise, reread the preceding material.

SUMMARY

Asian Americans and Pacific Islanders need specific, flexible treatment with emphasis on knowledge of their subcultures and acceptance of their different values. We have made generalizations about Asian Americans and Pacific Islanders and highlighted their emphasis on the family, extended kinship ties, respectful attitudes toward parents and other authority figures, and the interdependency of Asian-American and Pacific-Islander peoples.

However, we would not want anything that we have said to exclude the possibility of specific, individualized treatment planning for Asian Americans, including those who may be acculturated and need treatment plans quite similar and comparable to the mental health treatment of majority Americans.

REFERENCES

Adler, J., Lord, M., Newhall, E. F., McGuire, S., & Coppola, V. The new immigrants. *Newsweek*, July 7, 1980, pp. 26–31.

Chien, C. P. Concluding remarks, transcultural psychopharmacology in depression: East and West. *Psychopharmacology Bulletin*, 1979, 15(4), 44–45.

Fung, D. S., Uchalik, D., Lo, S. N., Reece, S., & Lam, J. *Treatment of Asian patients: Side effects and compliance*. Paper presented at the meeting of the Second Pacific Congress of Psychiatry, Manila, Philippines, May 1980.

Georgotas, A., & Gershon, S. Lithium plasma levels. *Psychopharmacology Bulletin*, 1979, 15(4), 35–37.

Glassman, A., & Roose, S. Tricyclic antidepressant drug tolerance in Oriental and Occidental populations. *Psychopharmacology Bulletin*, 1979, 15(4), 41–44.

Honda, Y., & Suzuki, T. Transcultural pharmacokinetic study on lithium concentration in plasma and saliva. *Psychopharmacology Bulletin*, 1979, 15(4), 37–39.

Kinsey, J. A summary of literature on epidemiology of mental illness in Hawaii. In W. S. Tseng, J. F. McDermott, Jr., & T. W. Maretzki (Eds.), *Peoples and cultures in Hawaii*. Honolulu: University of Hawaii Press, 1974.

Legge, J. The doctrine of the mean. Book three. In Confucius *The four books*. Taipei, Taiwan: Wen Yuen, 1973.

Mochizuki, M. *Discharge and units of service by ethnic origin: Fiscal year 1973–1974* (Vol. 3, Report No. 11). In Los Angeles County Department of Health Services, *E & R rows and columns*. Los Angeles: County of Los Angeles Department of Health Services, Mental Health Services, 1975.

President's Commission on Mental Health. *Report to the President* (Vol. 1). Washington, D.C.: U.S. Government Printing Office, 1978.

Schofield, W. *Psychotherapy: The purchase of friendship*. Englewood Cliffs, N.J.: Prentice-Hall, 1964.

Sue, S. Community mental health services to minority groups: Some optimism, some pessimism. *American Psychologist*, 1977, 32, 616–624.

Sue, S., & Sue, D. W. MMPI comparisons between Asian–Americans and non-Asian students utilizing a student health psychiatric clinic. *Journal of Counseling Psychology*, 1974, 21, 423–427.

Sue, S., & McKinney, H. Asian Americans in the community mental health system. *American Journal of Orthopsychiatry*, 1975, 45, 111–118.

Takahashi, R. *Lithium treatment of affective disorder in therapeutic plasma levels*. Paper presented at the meeting of the American College of Neuropsychopharmacology, Maui, Hawaii, December 1978.

Yamamoto, J. Psychotherapy for Asian Americans. In *The Second Pacific Congress of Psychiatry, Korea Extension Meeting 1980*. Seoul, Korea: The Korean Neuropsychiatric Assoc., May 1980.

Yamamoto, J., Fung, D., Lo, S., & Reece, S. Psychopharmacology for Asian Americans and Pacific Islanders. *Psychopharmacology Bulletin*, 1979, 15(4), 29–31.

Yamamoto, J., & Steinberg, A. Affect among Asian Americans. *Journal of the American Academy of Psychoanalysis*, 1981, 9(3), 447–457.

Yamashita, I., & Asano, Y. Tricyclic antidepressants: Therapeutic plasma level. *Psychopharmacology Bulletin*, 1979, 15(4), 40–41.

CHAPTER 7

Putting It All Together

Leonard A. Evans, Frank X. Acosta, and Joe Yamamoto

INTRODUCTION

Psychotherapy for the poor, working class, and minority patient requires a two-pronged thrust to be effective. First, therapists must be aware of the special characteristics which these patients bring to therapy, and second, the patients must be made more aware of what to expect from therapy and what is expected of them during therapy in order to improve results.

The first six chapters of this book have been directed at the therapist; this concluding chapter will focus on a patient-orientation program and how we have brought both the therapist and the patient programs together within a research project to improve services in our clinic.

PATIENT-ORIENTATION PROGRAM

In order to have the greatest impact on low-income and minority patients, we prepared a patient-orientation program for the purpose of assisting patients to understand mental health services more fully, identify their problems more clearly and be more open and assertive with their therapists. Unlike previous programs designed for more middle-class white Americans, our new multifaceted patient-orientation program provides an introduction to and a general explanation of behaviors which are desirable during psychotherapy. It does not prepare the patient for a particular type of therapy, for example, individual or group therapy, but rather is designed to generalize to many psychotherapeutic approaches. The specific objectives of the program are to enable patients who are about to experience psychotherapy for the first time to

1. Better understand the process of seeing a therapist
2. More clearly express problems, needs and therapy expectations to the therapist
3. Be more open, direct, assertive, and self-disclosing with the therapist
4. Take a more active role in the therapy process

The major component of the program is a slide/cassette program which contains the necessary information to enable patients to accomplish stated objectives. Additional program components provide an opportunity for patients to demonstrate their knowledge by completing a Knowledge Questionnaire, state their attitudes concerning psychotherapy by completing an Attitude Questionnaire, and to demonstrate the desired behavior in a simulated role-play situation. In the role play, patients are asked to practice assertive behaviors which they have just learned with a research team member simulating a therapist.

The slide/cassette program is entitled "Tell It Like It Is." This program was intended for people from a wide range of ethnic, language, and cultural backgrounds. Therefore, simple, concrete language and graphic characterizations were used liberally to enable divergent patient groups to identify with the information more easily.

On the basis of identified ethnic and cultural patient characteristics and needs, seven specific "ideas" or types of behavior were identified which, in the opinion of the authors, patients needed to demonstrate more frequently if therapy was to be more effective.

In all phases of the program's development, input was sought from both staff and patients. Thus, patients, psychologists, psychiatrists, psychiatric social workers, psychiatric residents, psychology interns, psychiatric nurses and community aides all contributed to establishing both the face validity and content validity of the program. Several versions of script dialogue and media were developed and reviewed. Reactions from patients gave us feedback on the impact and clarity of the information presented in the program. Care was taken to include in the program examples of problems and symptoms most common to patients in a public mental health facility, for example, depression, anxiety, interpersonal family problems, and sexual problems.

"Tell It Like It Is" begins with a brief narrated explanation of what psychotherapy is, and what a therapist does. This narration is illustrated by cartoons. The patients are then encouraged to ask questions freely of therapists or staff members. The seven ideas or suggested behaviors to use in therapy are then explained sequentially.

Each idea, and an accompanying key cartoon slide, is presented and followed by a vignette, which is illustrated with slides of actors portraying a patient–therapist dialogue which models the desired patient behavior. The patient and therapist actors used for the vignettes represent a cross-section of ethnic backgrounds, ages, and sexes. Ethnic groups most represented are Hispanic, black, and white. The dialogues vary for each vignette and capture ethnic voice differences. For each vignette, multiple patient–therapist scenes are shown in sequence with the dialogue.

For example, one of the ideas presented in the program is the need for patients to tell their therapists what is bothering them, even if it makes them feel uncomfortable or embarrassed. This is followed by a vignette of a male patient hesitantly telling his male therapist about the embarrassment he feels when he talks about sex. The patient then says that he thinks he has a problem but finds it really hard to talk about. The therapist in turn acknowledges the patient's difficulty in expressing his problem, explains that they must talk about the problem in order to solve it, and encourages further discussion.

Following each vignette, the idea being illustrated is briefly reviewed, along with its key cartoon, before proceeding to the next idea. At the end of the entire program, all seven suggested behaviors are again briefly reviewed in both the narration and the key cartoons.

Each patient is permitted to practice the assertiveness suggested by "Tell It Like It Is" prior to seeing a therapist. In the role-play situation, a research assistant describes a hypothetical scene in therapy and asks the patient to act out what is described. For example, the following scene is described:

> Imagine this is during your first visit with your therapist, which you will be going to in a few minutes. You have been talking with your therapist about 40 minutes and your session is coming to an end. Your therapist says he wants to see you once a week for eight or nine months, but you

think that you will be feeling better in much less time. You must then
explain to me, your therapist, that you have a different view in mind,
and explain how long you think you should come.

At this point the patient is encouraged and helped to practice an
assertive response.

A colorful reminder brochure has been designed and produced
to supplement the slide show. The brochure, which is available in
English and Spanish, uses selected cartoons and messages from "Tell
It Like It Is" to reinforce ideas presented in the program (see script
that follows for selected cartoons). Patients are encouraged to take
the brochure home and to refer to it between therapy sessions.

All these procedures and materials have been designed and used
in such a way that patients are better prepared to engage in a fruitful
psychotherapy session with their therapist.

THERAPIST-ORIENTATION PROGRAM

The primary aims of the therapist training program are to increase
the therapists' knowledge, sensitivity, and effectiveness in treating
low-income and minority patients, to increase positive responses to
patient assertiveness, to increase responsiveness and action to patient
requests and problems, and to increase the number of patients discharged as having received sufficient services. We attempted to
achieve these aims by developing a Minority Issues Seminar. There,
therapists discuss issues and information as presented in the preceding chapters, as well as their own experiences and feelings in treating
minority and low-income patients. Additional materials used include
relevant articles, slide shows such as "Tell It Like It Is," and films
portraying important characteristics of the white working class, Hispanic, black, and Asian Americans. Role-playing of specific therapist–minority patient issues is used throughout the seminar.

IMPACT OF THE PROGRAMS

The Minority Issues Seminar has been received with considerable
enthusiasm. Dialogue has been open and frank, and regular attendance has been high. Thus far, written postseminar evaluations have

been conducted for one class of psychology interns and for two classes of psychiatric residents. Initial analysis of the information suggests: (1) that patients are willing to be self-disclosing and assertive after participating in the patient-orientation program, and that they learned information about psychotherapy during the course of the program; and (2) therapists feel more knowledgeable about social class and cultural factors in therapy after being in the orientation seminar and reading the written material.

The effects of the patient- and therapist-orientation programs have significant implications for the delivery of mental health services both in the clinic where they were developed and throughout the country. This project is using innovative approaches with both patients and therapists. It is hoped that the study will show significant treatment benefit for patients who are oriented with a relatively brief and simple program. Such an orientation should help all patients receive better, more relevant services. Results to date have shown that a brief orientation can lead to increased information about psychotherapy and more positive attitudes toward it on the part of low-income and minority outpatients.

This study promises to contribute valuable information on the effects of patient preparation for treatment, sociocultural training of therapists, patient–therapist interactions, and cross-cultural factors among Hispanic, black, Asian, and white patients in both the process and outcome stages of treatment. This work is highly congruent with the objectives of the 1978 President's Commission on Mental Health Report, which strongly advocates increasing mental health services for the minority and poor.

SCRIPT FOR "TELL IT LIKE IT IS"

NARRATOR: The program you are going to see has seven ideas which can help you to get more out of being here. This program will present each idea and then show you pictures of people using that idea to help solve their problems of living and problems with feelings.

All people have some problems at various times in their lives, such as losing a job, or getting a divorce, which can cause stress, tension, or depression. Sometimes people feel physically sick even though doctors can find nothing wrong and say that their body is O.K.

Today, you will see someone who has special experience in helping people with problems of living and problems with feelings. The person you will see is called a therapist and the way you are helped is called therapy.

Therapy involves talking about yourself, your problems, and your feelings so that, with the help of your therapist, you can feel better.

If you do as this program advises and "tell it like it is" you will get more help and greater benefits from your therapy.

You will probably have some questions before you start your therapy.

So whenever you come here, feel free to ask the staff any questions you may have. Now, let's consider the first idea.

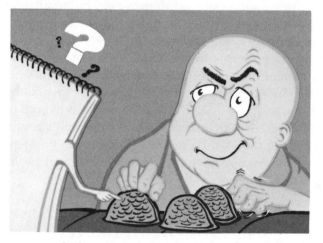

Try not to hide your problems. Your therapist won't know what you're thinking and feeling unless you "tell it like it is." Your therapist is only human, not a mind reader. So say how you feel, what you think your problems are, and what kind of help you want.

THERAPIST (White Man): It's hard for me to know what's troubling you. I wish you would tell me. You haven't told me exactly how you feel.

PATIENT (White Woman): Well (*pause*) . . . umm . . . (*pause*) . . . I came here because I feel awful. I want you to help me feel better.

THERAPIST: I'm glad you told me that. I do want to help. Could you tell me what you mean by awful?

PATIENT: Well, I cry a lot, and I'm nervous and upset all the time. You see, well, my husband and I are not getting along. It's not the same anymore. We don't talk to each other.

THERAPIST: I can see why you are upset. That does help me. Could you tell me more about it?

NARRATOR: Remember, don't hide your problems. Your therapist can only help you if you say what is wrong and explain what your problems are.

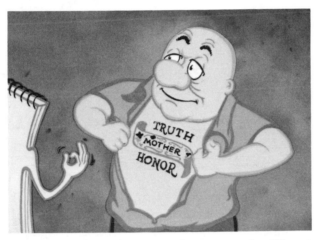

Our next idea is to be open, honest, and willing to express how you feel about anything, even about your therapist; for example. . . .

Don't be afraid to disagree with your therapist. What you think and feel are very important to you and to your therapist.

PATIENT (Chicana Woman): I know you're trying to help, but I'm not getting the help I want. You just seem to "uh-huh" all the time. I feel I'm not getting anywhere.

THERAPIST (Black Woman): Okay, thanks for telling me. Could you tell me what you expect from me?

PATIENT: I think you should tell me what to do. I came here with a problem, and I want you to take care of it!

THERAPIST: Well, I want to help you but I can't make problems disappear. We have to work together to solve them. Now, let's see what we can do about your problems. Let's go over the main one again.

PATIENT: Again? . . . Well, okay. My mother and I scream and yell at each other all the time. We just can't seem to agree on anything anymore . . .

NARRATOR: Remember, it is very imporant that you be open and honest with your therapist, and don't be afraid to disagree with your therapist. Your therapist is trying to help you.

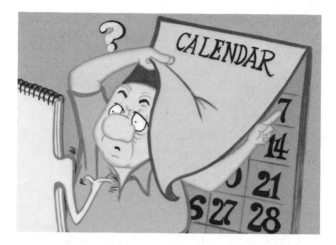

Another idea to consider is that, if you think your therapist is going to be treating you for too long a period of time, tell your therapist. Sometimes people expect to get better right away. Usually this doesn't happen. It may take a little more time to solve your problems than you had planned.

PATIENT (Chicano Man): I've been here three times and haven't solved my problems yet. I usually don't see the doctors this many times.

THERAPIST (White Man): I appreciate your telling me about it. But you know, some problems take a little more time than others.

Were you expecting to have your problems solved by now?

PATIENT: Well, I think that after seeing you for three times, I should have solved a couple of my problems. You know, like why am I still feeling so depressed and why do I still feel like I'm getting nowhere in my job.

NARRATOR: Remember, tell your therapist if you're not satisfied with the time it's taking to solve your problems.

A fourth idea is that, if you don't plan on coming back for your next appointment, whatever the reason is, say so.

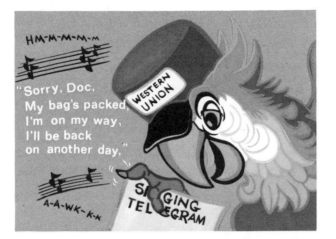

PATIENT (Black Man): You know, I've been feeling a lot better for the
last month. I don't think I need to come back to therapy anymore.

THERAPIST (White Man): I'm glad to hear that you're feeling better.
Could you tell me more about how you feel?

PATIENT: Well, I feel you've helped me understand myself. I think I
can handle my problems better now.

THERAPIST: Well, you've made a lot of progress. I agree with you, I
don't think you have to come back anymore. But, if you ever do
have problems again, please call and let me know.

NARRATOR: Remember, no matter what the reason is, good or bad, tell
your therapist if you don't plan on coming back for your next
appointment.

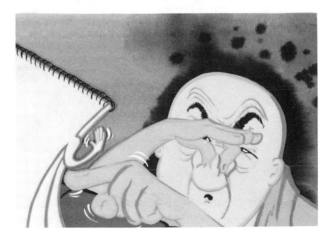

Idea number five: If, for some reason, you're unhappy with your therapist, tell your therapist. You have a right to think and feel as you do.

PATIENT (White Woman): I don't like coming here, it's too hard. (*On the verge of tears*) I don't feel you're helping me that much . . .

THERAPIST (Chicano Man): I'm sorry you feel that way. I can see it was hard for you to say that . . . (*pause*) Can you tell me more about how you feel?

PATIENT: Well, since I've been coming here, I've been trying really hard, but I still feel nervous.

I have trouble falling asleep, and I wake up too early. My stomach still burns. I should be well by now.

THERAPIST: I know you're still hurting. But I don't think meeting here five times is enough to change the pains you've developed over several years.

I think you can benefit if we continue to discuss your problems just a few more times.

NARRATOR: Remember, tell your therapist if you're unhappy with your therapy. They can only help you if you say how you feel. Your therapist wants to help you.

Talking about certain problems may make you feel awkward, or embarrassed. Our next idea is that:

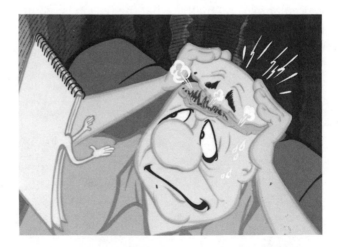

You should talk about your problems, even though it may make you feel uncomfortable. Talking about them will probably help.

THERAPIST (White Man): I've noticed that you get really tense whenever you talk about sex.

PATIENT (White Man): Yeah, well, I . . . (*long silence . . . 5 seconds*) I just feel real embarrassed when I talk about sex, you know.

THERAPIST: Is it just with me, or anyone?

PATIENT: Anyone, I guess. I think I have a problem. But I just can't tell you what's wrong. It's really hard to talk about, you know.

THERAPIST: I can see it's difficult for you. Is this a problem you'd like to work on? If it is, we have to talk about it.

PATIENT: Well . . . I do want to solve my problem.

NARRATOR: Remember, even though talking about certain problems may make you feel embarrassed and uncomfortable, you should talk to your therapist about these problems so that your therapist can help you solve them.

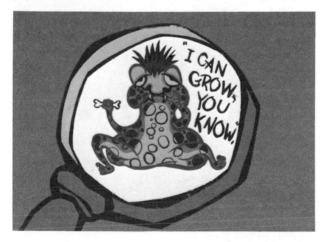

Our last idea is that you can talk to your therapist about any problem you may be having. For example: work, money, sex, personal feelings, welfare, medical, family, school, or anything, whether you are seen by your therapist individually or in a group.

No problem is too small to talk about. Sometimes even little things, if left unattended, can become major problems.

PATIENT (Black Woman): I hate to bother you with this little problem, but I keep waking up early in the morning and just can't get back to sleep.

THERAPIST (White Man): Well, let's see. Your waking up might be important. Has anything in particular been troubling you this week?

PATIENT: Well, I hadn't thought about it, but I have felt pretty low lately (*tears . . . softly*)

THERAPIST: It's good you brought this up. Let's try to figure out what's been making you feel low.

NARRATOR: Remember, no matter how small your problems may seem to you, they may be very important, so tell your therapist.

   The seven ideas and examples you have just seen about therapy were to help you tell it like it is. By using them, you will get more help and greater benefits from your therapy, whether you see a therapist by yourself, or in a group. Now, let's briefly review the seven ideas.

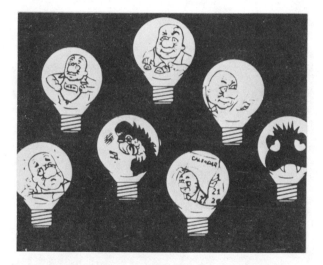

   One, don't hide your problems.

   Two, be open, honest, and willing to express how you feel, even if it means disagreeing with your therapist.

   Three, if you think your therapist is going to be treating you for too long a period of time, let your therapist know.

   Four, if you don't plan on coming back for your next appointment, no matter what the reason is, tell your therapist.

   Five, if you are happy, or unhappy, with your therapy, tell your therapist.

   Six, even if you feel uncomfortable or embarrassed about certain problems, talk to your therapist about them.

   Seven, feel free to talk about any problems you may have.

   No problem is too small.

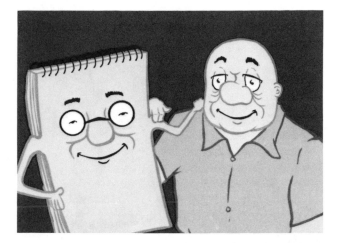

Remember, these seven ideas are only examples of things which may help you in your therapy. Therapists are here to try to help you with your own special problems. It's what you think and feel that's important. So . . . tell it like it is.

REFERENCES

President's Commission on Mental Health. *Report to the President* (Vol. 1). Washington, D.C.: U.S. Government Printing Office, 1978.

Index